COUPLE

WORKBOOK

What a husband and wife need to do to fix their marriage.
Resolve conflicts and build deep connections before
your relationship falls apart

JANIS BRYANS PSY.D

TABLE OF CONTENTS

INTRODUCTION

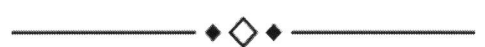

Relationships are not easy. They require regular maintenance and work if they are to continue to prosper and grow. Perhaps you have found the person you want to spend your life with. At first, your relationship may have been full of joy and love, and you wanted to spend every waking moment with your partner. In this bliss of new love, everything may well have felt perfect.

But as our lives progress and we grow as people, it can lead to tension between ourselves and our partners. Do you feel as though, these days, you and your partner spend most of your time together arguing? Does it feel as though you can't even agree on what to eat for dinner, let alone major decisions such as where to live or how to raise your children?

If so, you're not alone. When the gloss of a new relationship has worn off and we are faced with the challenges life throws at us, it can put a strain on our relationship.

No doubt you are reading this because you want to strengthen your marriage, or relationship. Picking up this book is an important first step. It sends a signal to yourself that you are willing to make changes in order to save your partnership – in other words, by picking up this book you are affirming that your relationship is important to you, and very much worth saving.

For many couples, when they face challenges in their relationship, they seek the help of a marriage counsellor. And while this book is not intended as a replacement for face to face couples therapy, it can assist you in identifying and clarifying difficulties in your relationship and offer methods of working through them with your partner.

Even if you are not facing challenges in your marriage, this book can also be of use. It will guide you on best practices for strengthening your relationship and ensuring you and your partner remain happy and connected long into the future.

We will examine overarching issues such as

- What you should and shouldn't be doing if you want to save your marriage
- How to avoid and remove the behaviors that can damage your relationship
- Communication techniques that will assist in strengthening your relationship

In Part One, we will delve into exactly what constitutes a relationship, including an examination of the different types of love, and the characteristics of different couplings. We will also take a look at some of the challenges couples face, and common traits of successful couples, including behaviors to both adopt and avoid.

Part Two will delve deeper into some of the issues faced by couples including financial disagreements, misaligned personal values and a struggling sex life. It will also examine some of the challenges faced by specific couplings, such as young couples, or couples with a significant age gap. Though exercises and suggestions, we will examine ways to resolve these important and common issues.

Part Three will look closely at what to expect in the event that you decide to pursue therapy with a licensed relationship counsellor.

Fixing a broken relationship is not easy, but the rewards are immense. It is my hope that this book will inspire you first to believe that your marriage can be saved, and secondly, to be willing to make the necessary changes. Practicing the exercises in this book will help you to remember exactly why you and your partner fell in love in the first place and will strengthen your bond so you can face the challenges of life together.

The work will not always be easy, but it will be worth it.

PART ONE:

UNDERSTANDING RELATIONSHIPS

CHAPTER ONE: DIFFERENT TYPES OF RELATIONSHIPS – WHAT'S YOURS?

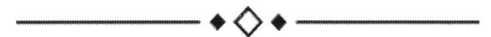

As humans, our lives are full of many different relationships, and – if we are lucky – many different types of love. But love is such a broad and often intangible concept that it is impossible to really define. Throughout our lifetimes, we will likely experience many different types of love, including the unconditional love a parent has a for a child and the affectionate love we have for our friends. If we are lucky, we will also experience self-love, often a difficult thing to find.

But the focus of this book is romantic love, also known by the ancient Greco-Christian term *eros*. This is the love shared by two members of a couple; the type of love we are aiming to rekindle, build or save when we enter couples therapy.

But if we look closer at romantic love, we discover that this too can be divided into a number of different facets. To examine this further, let's take a look at the Triangular Theory of Love, a theory put forth by psychologist Robert J. Sternberg, of Cornell University.

The Triangular Theory of Love

Recognizing the kind of love you and your partner share is a crucial first step in understand your relationship – and overcoming difficulties you face as a couple. In 1985, Sternberg put forth a theory outlining seven different types of love, entitled the Triangular Theory of Love.

This theory proposes that most human relationships contain a mix of three elements: passion, intimacy and commitment. While a relationship can exist featuring just one of these elements, more often, it is a combination of these three elements that produce the more complex loving relationships that we as humans actively seek.

According to Sternberg's theory, when two of these three elements can combine in different formats, each time producing a different kind of love. For example, intimacy combined with commitment forms companionate love, passion plus intimacy equals romantic love and commitment combined with passion equals fatuous love. Each of these three love types form one side of the triangular diagram that gives this theory its name.

But what happens when all three of these love types are combined? This, according to Sternberg, produces consummate love, which is often seen as the ideal for which all couples strive. A couple sharing consummate love enjoys all three elements: passion, intimacy and commitment, and the result is a happy, long-lasting and secure relationship.

This consummate love should be the goal for all couples – and it is the goal of this book to help you and your partner reach or rekindle that feeling. The exercises in the coming chapters are all based around improving either passion, intimacy or commitment – sometimes a combination of two or three – paving the way for an increased sense of connection.

The Five Relationship Types

While consummate love is an ideal for which many of us strive, the reality is that too few couples are able to achieve this goal. If you have picked up this book, your relationship is likely lacking in one of the three key areas.

It can be very useful on your journey towards a happy, loving relationship to identify exactly where your relationship is now; in other words, to identify your starting point. The personality traits and underlying issues of both yourself and your partner play an important role in determining what kind of couple you make. You and your partner's propensity for domination or submissiveness, your need for approval and your typical response to conflict are all elements that determine the type of coupling you produce. While these elements can of course be changed, knowing your strengths and weaknesses as individuals and as a couple gives you a great starting point for growth and change.

With that in mind, let's take a look at the five most common types of couplings:

Type One: The Active/Passive Couple

In this type of coupling, one of the partners is dominant. The person in charge makes the majority of the decisions, while the other partner simply goes with the flow. Most often, this relationship dynamic will have been present from the beginning, with the active partner choosing to adopt a "caretaker" role. Often, a partner who takes on this role has spent their lifetime pleasing others and taking on responsibilities that are not necessarily their own. In contrast, the passive partner often has a history of anxiety and becomes easily overwhelmed.

This type of coupling can also be the result of external situations such as illness or physical trauma: in such a situation, one partner is forced to step up and become the active partner in the relationship, effectively taking on a caretaker role.

While this coupling does not often lead to regular arguments, the active partner can sometimes be prone to resentment and outbursts if they feel as though they do not receive enough gratitude and appreciation for their work.

Long term, active/passive couples risk the active partner becoming resentful and burned out.

Type Two: The Aggressive/Accommodating Couple

Just like in the active/passive coupling, this relationship type is also typified by an imbalance of power. In this case, however, the difference comes about not due to one partner taking on a caretaker role, but rather seeking to exert power over the other. In such a coupling, one partner is clearly dominant, with the other acting passively often out of fear. Such relationships often involve emotional and/or physical abuse.

Often the aggressive partner in such a coupling will suffer from anger management issues, and will often have grown up with an abusive caregiver. They may also suffer from anxiety which manifests itself in a need for control and lack of empathy.

Interestingly, the passive partner may also have suffered an abusive childhood, with the difference that they have simply developed a tolerance for such behavior. Often, such partners believe that if they treat their aggressive partner well, they will be rewarded with their partner's sporadic kindness.

Aggressive/accommodating relationships rarely end with the aggressive partner walking away. Rather, these relationships will simply continue unchanged, on the passive partner will find the strength to end the coupling. As a result, the aggressive partner will seek to lure them back into the relationship or will find someone else to fulfil the passive role.

Type Three: The Competitive/Controlling Couple

This type of relationship is also about power, but in this case, the couple is in regular conflict in order to determine who is dominant. This type of couple is typified by two strong personalities who constantly challenge each other over who is right or wrong, or whose way is better. This is tense relationship type, in which couples strive constantly to have the last word.

People in this relationship type often feel the need to win their battles as a matter of self-esteem and see winning as the be all and end all, regardless of how detrimental it may be to the relationship.

Competitive/controlling couples often end in divorce or separation, or, more optimistically, they develop the ability to mark their own claims on areas in their lives for which they will individually take responsibility.

Type Four: The Disconnected/Parallel Lives Couple

This type of relationship, couples rarely argue, but nor do they rarely connect. To all intents and purposes, they live their own independent lives, as they often have little in common. Often, people in this type of coupling can feel more like housemates than lovers. A disconnected coupling can create a cold home environment, with the relationship feeling stale, despite the partners' courteousness to each other.

Usually, this type of relationship develops over a number of years, with the initial spark of romance quickly fading. Such couples may have married for the wrong reasons, or come up against insurmountable differences that they chose to push aside rather than face. Conversation can be a struggle in such a relationship, with small talk about topics like the weather, or updates on their children's lives being the go-to subjects of conversation.

Often, such coupling end when one of both partners decides that "life to too short" to continue in a relationship that is devoid of passion. Alternatively, they may decide to simply settle, rationalizing that what they have is good enough, or they are simply too old or set in their ways to make a change.

Type Five: The Accepting/Balanced Couple

While the four types of relationships above are destructive in their various ways, the following relationship type is seen as the ideal. It is the type of coupling we ought to strive for – and the goal of many who attend couples therapy.

In an accepting/balanced relationship, there is no power struggle, with both partners able to work effectively as a team. They are aware of each other's strengths and weaknesses and do their best to support each other when they can. Such couples are able to confront any problems they may face in their relationship and do their best to improve the situation when needed.

While such couples inevitably have moments of conflict, they are able to work through these in a calm, respectful and understanding manner. The accepting/balanced couple is the couple most likely to stay together, working through life's challenges together in a loving way.

While many relationships are accepting and balanced from the beginning, couples in any of the other four relationship types are also able to reach this desired state. Through self-analysis and therapy, they can make the necessary changes in order to make their relationship stronger and healthier.

Can you see features of your own relationship in any of these five types? Reread each description carefully and, as honestly as you can, see if you can identify any of the above behaviors as your own. Remember, being able to identify the type of coupling you are in provides a firm starting point for building and improving your relationship.

Exercises:

CHAPTER TWO: BEHAVIORS THAT CAN KILL YOUR RELATIONSHIPS

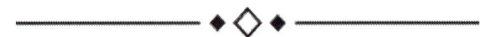

Take a moment to step back and think carefully about your relationship. If you have picked up this book, it's likely there are a number of areas in which you can improve.

Perhaps you know exactly what is causing the friction between you and your partner. Maybe there is an issue in your lives on which you cannot agree. Or perhaps your marriage seems to just be one argument after another, with no evident underlying cause.

If your relationship is facing difficulties, there are likely to be a number of different behaviors that contribute to the conflict. Some of these might be major disagreements, while others are everyday actions we may not even be aware are causing conflict.

Let's take a look at some of the most common habits that can damage – or even kill – our relationships.

Constantly criticizing ourselves and pointing out our flaws.

When we suffer from low self-esteem, we often fall into a pattern of self-criticism that is so second nature we barely realize we are doing it. But the truth is, more often than not, the only person who notices these flaws is yourself. Remember, your partner chose to be with you for your good traits, and he or she sees these features, even if you can't see them yourself.

But when you focus on your flaws – constantly pointing out your inability to say the right thing, or the fact that you keep burning dinner, or those few extra pounds you've put on – it can do damage to your relationship. When you constantly criticize yourself this way, you are sending a message to your partner that you are not happy, and it can become easy for your loved one to blame themselves for this.

Conversely, when you constantly point out your flaws, they can begin to override the good traits that your partner had once focused on, and you might eventually convince your partner to see you in the same negative way that you see yourself.

Trying to be the perfect partner

None of us are perfect, and we are only deluding ourselves if we try to be. Sure, it may be that you love your partner so much that you want to do everything for them; clean the house, make dinner, do the laundry, earn enough to support you both… the list can be endless. But as well-meaning as this habit may seem, trying to be the perfect partner can lead to resentment as you realize you cannot possibly maintain this image of perfection. Similarly, when you try and do everything for your partner, you are denying them the chance to be self-sufficient and independent, which is an important element when it comes to building a secure relationship.

Being judgmental and negative

It doesn't matter how much affection and love you lavish on your partner; when you are bitter and judgmental towards the rest of the world, it can have a damaging effect on your relationship. When you view the world through a negative lens – and make a habit of sharing these thoughts – you infuse your space with negative energy, dragging down those around you; in this case, your partner. Such negative energy can cause your partner to also see the worst; both in the relationship, and the world around you.

Not valuing your partner's opinion

This can be a challenge for those of us who are particularly strong-minded, or who have been single for a long period of time. In such situations, it can be easy to convince ourselves that we are always right, and that it is not important to listen to the opinions of our partner. But of course, such behavior can be very damaging in a relationship. For a relationship to grow and prosper, it must be based on mutual respect and understanding; and a big part of this is listening to what your partner has to say. Even if your partner's opinion differs to your own, take time to listen to what that have to say without passing judgement or getting frustrated or angry. See any disagreements as an opportunity to learn more about each other and strengthen your relationship through compromise and understanding. We will be examining how to manage conflicts with respect and composure later in this book.

Overspending

In many cases, conflict within a relationship is caused by disagreements over money. Overspending habits can put particular strain on relationships, as can a reluctance to talk openly about the issue or overtightening the purse strings. Understanding your partner's money handling habits, beliefs, fears and goals are crucial to avoiding conflict in this area. We will be discussing conflict around financial issues in detail in Chapter Nine.

Comparing your partner to others

Comparing your partner to a former lover can be a natural thing to do, but when comparisons take place regularly, they can cause damage to a relationship. Of course, when you negatively compare your partner to others, it can be very destructive to their self-esteem, but it is important to note than favorably comparing your partner to past relationships can be similarly damaging. Each time you refer back to a prior relationship, you send your partner a message that you are living in the past – that your ex is still in your mind. Instead of focusing on things that no longer are, embrace the present with your loved one.

Drawing comparisons can also go further than assessing your partner against former lovers. Learn to become aware of any throwaway lines you use that compare your spouse to others in your life. These could be seemingly innocuous comments such as "When Mom used to make this dish, she put more cheese on top" or "My best friend has a better taste in movies than you." Such comments can be damaging to your partner's self-esteem if they build up over time, causing cracks to appear in your relationship.

Dwelling on past mistakes

Similarly, another damaging behavior is dwelling on past mistakes. If you keep count and linger on your partner's errors and faults, it is likely to lead to fresh conflict. In addition, when you dwell on a mistake instead of confronting and solving it, you run the risk of bottling up your negative emotions which can lead to bigger problems in the future.

Giving subtle hints instead of being direct

Likely, we've all been here at one point or another. Your partner has upset you, and when they ask what's wrong, you simply murmur "nothing,", then sigh and walk away. We do this in the hope that our partner will realize their mistake and come to their senses. But the reality is, dropping hints like this, rather than openly expressing your feelings, rarely gets the message across. Sure, your partner might pick up that you are upset, but will likely struggle to determine exactly why, making it impossible for them to fix any mistakes they may have made. Even in the most trusting and loving relationships, we cannot expect our partners to read our minds. Dropping hints rather than openly expressing our disappointment or anger sends a signal to your partner that you are not able to be honest and upfront with them or are unwilling to take responsibility for your words.

Trying to make your partner jealous

We often do this when we feel we are not getting enough attention from our partner or are feeling underappreciated. But when we try to punish our partner by making them feel jealous, we are undermining the security of our relationship.

Forcing your partner to say I love you

Hearing "I love you" from the right person can bring us endless amounts of joy. But the phrase loses its meaning when we goad someone into saying it. Expressions of love should be given spontaneously, without prompting, or else they run the risk of feeling forced, insincere or routine. If you find yourself constantly asking your partner if they love you, take a moment to consider why you are engaging in this behavior. Likely, it is a sign that you feel insecure in the relationship, which is a concern you should raise with your partner.

Spending too much time on your phone

In today's day and age, it is all too easy to get caught up in social media, the news, or the latest sporting results. We find ourselves constantly checking our phones, often instinctively, without truly feeling the need. But when you and your partner spend your time "together" glued to your phone screens, it causes a disconnect in the relationship. Particularly if you have children, and/or a busy work schedule, alone time can be precious and rare. Ensure you put your phones away and give each other your full attention.

Constantly threatening to leave

For some of us, our instinctive reaction to troubles in a relationship can be to make threats to leave. We may use this as ammunition when we are losing a fight or facing a seemingly insurmountable issue. And yes, there may well be times when leaving is the right response (particularly if any kind of abuse is present.) But if you are truly invested in a relationship, and as simply using this threat as a bargaining tool, it can cause endless damage to your relationship. By threatening to leave, you are sending a signal to your partner that you do not necessarily value your relationship – that it is easier to walk away than to invest time in fixing what you have built.

Needing to know everything about where your partner has been

One of traits of healthy relationships is that each partner has their own life outside of the coupling. To allow your relationship to grow and strengthen, it is important that you allow your partner to have his or her own interests and friends. Refrain from asking your loved one for every detail of time spent apart. When you do this, you are suggesting that you do not trust them, and may come across as controlling and paranoid. By all means, show an active interest in your loved one's life, but do so when they offer information on their own accord, rather than hounding it out of them.

Exercises:

CHAPTER THREE: THE HABITS OF SUCCESSFUL COUPLES

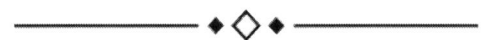

Do you find yourself going through a string of failed relationships, while those around you all seem to be happy and content in their marriages? Do you ever stop to wonder what they are doing differently? Perhaps you have now found yourself with a partner you feel you could build a future with and want to do your best to make things last.

We have taken at look at behavioral traits that can damage relationships, but what about the behaviors that strengthen them? What are the secrets of those couples who have made their relationships last for twenty, thirty, forty years or longer? Is it simply a case of learning to put up with your partner's challenging behaviors? Or is there much more to it?

Couples therapists agree there are a number of important traits present in successful relationships that all couples should aspire to. Let's take a look:

Forgiving one another

Developing the ability to forgive your partner freely is one of the most important skills to develop when it comes to improving our relationship.

But what exactly does it mean to forgive deeply and freely? Many of us have never stopped to consider exactly what forgiveness entails. We think of it as a vague concept of letting go of wrongs that were committed against us; forgetting and moving on. But true forgiveness is about far more than simply moving on. Real forgiveness involves not only letting go of the wrongs done to you, but replacing the hurt it caused with something positive, such as understanding, empathy, compassion and, in the case of our spouses, deep love.

Many of us have the incorrect belief that forgiving someone means allowing them to get away with whatever they did to us. But this is simply not the case. Forgiving someone does not mean we are not forgoing our need for justice, an apology, or reconciliation. Forgiveness is separate from the three things. For example, receiving an apology necessarily mean a person is forgiven. And forgiving a person does not mean we are obliged to reconcile with them. Forgiveness is a place we must come to independently of these three elements.

Another common misconception is that forgiveness is a sign of weakness, but this is simply not the case. True forgiveness can be immensely difficult to give and requires a great deal of inner strength. As I'm sure you will agree, this is as far from weakness as one can get.

Forgiveness can be considered as having two elements: decisional and emotional. Decisional forgiveness occurs when we consciously move from a place of ill will towards a person to wishing them well. We no longer wish for bad things to happen to the person who has hurt us an important first step on the journey. This is most often the easiest element of forgiveness to manage.

But emotional forgiveness goes much deeper. This type of forgiveness takes place when we are able to actively move away from the negative feelings the wrongdoing invoked in us and replace them with far more positive emotions. This part of forgiveness often takes time, as it is human nature to dwell on negative emotions and even when we feel we have moved on, they have a tendency to return when we least expect it. This is especially prevalent when our spouse has committed a major wrongdoing against us, such as telling lies or being unfaithful. Sometimes even the smallest trigger can lead us to recall events we thought we were over.

There are a number of reasons why we should develop the capacity to forgive. In all likelihood, you are aware of the link between stress and physical ailments. Anxiety, worry, and resentment is linked to a wide range of illnesses. Chronic anger puts us into a constant fight-or-flight mode, which causes changes in heart rate, blood pressure and immunity. Those changes increase the risk of depression, heart disease and diabetes, among other conditions. But the good news is that there are also links between forgiveness and improved mental and physical health. When we forgive, we are releasing the stress associated with our negative feelings which leads to reduced anxiety, depression and other mental illnesses.

Forgiving your partner for their wrongdoings also sends out a powerful message. When you do so, you are making them aware that you know they did not intentionally set out to hurt you, as there is love between the two of you. This is an important first step in letting your relationship mend.

Complimenting your partner

Regularly complimenting your partner is a simple way to show what you value in your loved one. It contributes to your spouse's positive self-esteem and provides a focus on all that it good about your relationship.

But while complimenting your partner when the two of you alone is great, the relationship can be further strengthened by making these positive comments in front of others. And this needn't be a showy, declaration of all that is wonderful about your spouse. Simple throwaway lines to friends and family such as "My husband made a great dinner last night" or "She always picks up the phone when I call" can go a long way to maintaining closeness and a sense of appreciation within a relationship.

Focusing on the positives

All relationships have their ups and downs, even the strongest and most loving ones. But for a relationship to be happy and successful, the positive moments must outweigh the negative. Successful couples make a habit of pointing out the positives within their relationship. They thank each other for kind words or actions, give compliments freely, and congratulate one another on their successes.

Similarly, couples tend to be stronger when they laugh a lot. This is a powerful trait that helps prevent life from becoming weighed down with stressors. Of course, all couples will face serious issues throughout their life, but being able to face challenges with a sense of humor can be a powerful asset.

Understanding each other's differences

Most often, the cracks that form in a relationship are the result of two clashing personality types. We can easily interpret our partner's behavior as an attempt to create conflict or start an argument. But more often than not, disagreements arise because different personalities approach situations indifferent ways. Something we see as just a normal part of our day-to-day behavior may drive our partner mad; for example, if one habitually messy partner fails to put their clothes away at the end of the day. The tidy partner might misconstrue this as their loved one deliberately being lazy or disrespectful, while for the messy partner, it was merely a subconscious reaction with no deeper motive.

Successful couples invest time in understanding who their partner is; what drives them, what irritates them, and what is important to them. When we develop a deeper understanding of our partner's inherent personality traits, we make it easier to avoid conflict, and to more effectively handle disagreements when they arise.

Expressing interest in one another's lives

While it's crucial that you and your partner have independent interests, one of the traits of successful couples is their ability to show interest in their partner's lives. This includes areas such as work life, friendships, family and hobbies. Ask questions regularly and listening intently to the answers.

This also goes a long way to assuring you partner that you are comfortable with the part of their life that you are not involved in.

Letting each other know when they will be home

Of course, in any healthy relationship there will be times when couples are apart. And one simple trait shared by many successful couples is that they consistently let their partner know when to expect them home. While it may seem petty or unnecessary, the simple act of calling or texting to let your partner know when you will be back helps build a sense of trust and security within a relationship and helps eliminate anxiety and worry.

Flirting with each other

Flirting is one of the keys to maintaining not only an active sex life, but also a connected and loving relationship outside the bedroom. Even – and especially – for couples who have been together for many years, flirting is a powerful way to show your attraction for your partner and keep the spark alive. When flirting is no longer present, the relationship runs the risk of becoming stale and mundane, both in and out of the bedroom.

Don't fight dirty

All couples fight, even the strongest ones. But those in successful relationships ensure that, when things get tense, they do not resort to name-calling, put downs, or digging up the past. Even when you and your partner disagree, respecting one another is key.

Developing both shared and individual interests

While successful couples have many things in common, they also have their own individual interests. To thrive as a couple, it is important to make time to develop shared hobbies and passions, but equally crucial to allow one another space to follow their own interests.

To develop your shared interests, think back to what drew you to your partner in the first place. In all likelihood, you are able to pinpoint a number of things you have in common, which can develop into shared hobbies – if they have not done so already. These interests can be as simple as watching a movie together, or as complex as accompanying each other on the trip of a lifetime. Sharing interests and hobbies with your partner allows you to connect in new ways and create fresh memories of your lives together.

And when it comes to individual interests, successful couples make room for each other's unique hobbies and passions. They show an interest in each other's passion, asking questions and actively listening to the answer.

Going to bed at the same time

Differences in schedules and sleeping patterns can make this a challenge for many couples. But to strengthen your relationship, try to make adjustments so you and your partner can go to bed at the same time several times a week. The act of falling asleep side by side, while experiencing skin-to-skin contact is incredibly effective at strengthening the bonds of a relationship.

Taking time to connect

In the previous chapter, we discussed the damage that can be wreaked on our relationship when we spend too much time glued to our mobile phones. Conversely, successful couples carve out time to truly connect, no matter how busy life gets, and no matter what is going on in the rest of the world – or on their social media feeds. These moments of connection can be as simple as going for a walk, chatting over dinner, or even doing the dishes together. It's not the activity that's important, rather it's the fact that you set aside specific time to be together.

Exercises:

PART TWO:
WORKING TO IMPROVE YOUR
RELATIONSHIP

CHAPTER FOUR: GETTING TO KNOW YOUR PARTNER

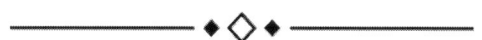

Take a moment to think about how well you really know your partner. Think about who they are at a fundamental level; do you know what drives your spouse to get out of bed each morning? What are their life goals? Their fears? What makes them happiest?

Perhaps, by asking yourself these questions, you may come to the realization that you know less about who your partner really is than you had initially believed. Perhaps you know everything about them on a superficial level but can't quite determine exactly what makes them tick.

Conversely, other couples may have been together for so long they feel as though they know everything there is to know about there spouse. It can feel as though there are no surprises left in the relationship; that your lives – and your partner themselves – have become predictable.

The reality is, even the longest and most enduring of relationships will never lead us to know everything about our partner. Human beings are complex creatures who are constantly changing. Often we find it difficult to truly understand what is going in our own minds. So how can we possibly understand what's going on in someone else's head when we can't even make sense of what's going on inside our own?

A large number of conflicts within relationships arise when couples simply do not understand each other. As we discussed in Chapter Two, some disagreements and problems can arise through simple misunderstandings, or personal values that are misconstrued as attempts at creating conflict. Getting to know your partner on a deeper level can help put an end to such misunderstandings. By understanding what is and isn't important to our partner, we begin to see their actions for what they truly are, rather than viewing them through the distorted lens of our own values and perceptions.

Beyond this, taking the time to really get to know your partner can help establish – or re-establish – closeness and connection within the relationship. It can serve as a timely reminder that, no matter how long you have been together, there is always something to learn about the person you have chosen to spend your life with.

The simplest way to get to know your partner is to ask questions. And "questions" here refers to deep, meaningful questions that do more than scratch the surface – not just the standard "how was your day?" that many couples routinely trot out each evening. Far too often, couples talk, but they do not actively share.

To truly know our partner, we must do more than merely engage in small talk. Psychology professor Dan Adams purports there are three different levels on which we can know a person; and to truly make a relationship work, we must endeavor to know our partner on all three of these levels:

Level One: General Characteristics and Personality Traits

Knowing a person on this level means we understand them in terms of their overarching personality. This includes whether they are introverted or extraverted, friendly, hard-working, open, or neurotic, along with other broad personality traits. Generally, we can get to know a person at this level through general conversation.

Level Two: Personal Values and Motivations

When we know a person on this second level, we are acquainted with their values, life goals and motivation. In other words, we understand what makes them tick. Knowledge at this level is acquired when we spend extended periods of time with a person, often through co-habitation or traveling together.

Level Three: Self-Narrative

According to Adams, the final level of knowing occurs when we understand a person in relation to their self-narrative; that is, we know the way they perceive themselves and how they make sense of the world around them. This is the most difficult of the levels to reach and is best done through a series of designed questions and discussion, such as the questions below.

Getting to Know Your Partner Through Questions

If you and your partner find it hard to move past small talk in your conversations – or if you are struggling to converse at all – these questions can be a helpful way of sparking discussion and opening up to one another. They take out the challenge of "finding something to talk about" and reduce the chance of falling to uncomfortable silences or resorting to superficial conversation.

You can make a game or event of it; putting time aside on a date night to really delve into what makes each other tick. These questions can address life's deeper issues or can be light-hearted and fun – often it is these seemingly whimsical questions that reveal the most about a person. While asking each other these questions, be sure to make eye contact to make it clear you have each other's full attention.

Let's take a look at a few suggestions.

Light-hearted questions to ask your partner

- What is your favorite song?
- What is your favorite book and why?
- What movie did you love as a child?
- What's your favorite memory with your mom/dad?
- Where have you always wanted to travel?
- Did you enjoy high school or college more?

- Describe the best party you've ever attended.
- What makes you most angry?
- What are you scared of?
- Did you collect anything as a child?
- Which of your friends would you choose to live on a desert island with?
- What would you do with a million dollars?
- Did you feel as though you fitted in as a child?
- If you could go back to any time in your life again, what would you choose?
- Did you ever rebel against your parents?
- Do you ever compare yourself to others?
- Which of my friends do you enjoy spending time with the most?
- What's your most unique talent?
- Who was your first crush?
- Describe your first kiss.
- What movie reminds you of our relationship?
- Do you prefer kissing or cuddling?
- When was the last time you cried?
- When was the last time you sang a song? Was it to yourself or someone else?
- If you could invite anyone to a dinner party, who would it be?
- What does a perfect day look like for you?
- Would you like to be famous? In what way?

Deeper Questions to Ask Your Partner:

- Which of your parents are you most like, and why?
- Do you ever dream about me?
- What is your sexual fantasy?
- When do you feel most safe and protected?
- Do you enjoy spending time with my friends? Why or why not?
- What did you learn about relationships from your parents and grandparents?

- Which partner before me had the greatest impact on you (positive or negative)?
- Do you believe in God?
- Which of your parents did you seek out when you were in trouble?
- What do you think of long-distance couples?
- Do you consider yourself an introvert or extravert?
- If you had to change one thing about yourself, what would it be?
- Do you consider yourself and optimist, pessimist or realist?
- How do you think you will die?
- If you could wake up tomorrow with one new ability or personality trait, what would it be?
- What do you consider your greatest accomplishment?
- What is your worst memory?
- Describe your relationship with your mother.
- What is your most embarrassing moment?
- What does love mean to you?
- What is too serious to be joked about?

You may choose to ask just one or two questions each, or a longer series of questions. Whatever you choose, allow your partner time to consider their answer, and do not interrupt them while they are speaking. Maintain eye contact as much as possible – this goes a long way towards building a deeper connection and trust.

You may find yourself surprised or taken aback by some of your partner's responses. Try to refrain from making any judgements. The goal here is not to create new areas of conflict within your relationship, but to open up to one another on a new and deeper level. If something your partner says elicits a negative response in you, take note of it and return to the discussion once the questioning is over. Express your thoughts and concerns in a calm and clear manner and allow your partner to respond in kind.

Exercises:

CHAPTER FIVE: CREATING A RELATIONSHIP VISION

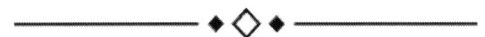

Challenges can arise within a relationship when the partners do not share a vision for the future. Their individual goals and desires lead them to move in different directions, putting a strain on the relationship and making it feel as though their lives are incompatible.

In order for a relationship to function successfully, both partners must have a vision for their future that aligns with one another. This is not to say that each party cannot have their own individual goals and aspirations for tomorrow – in fact, having a degree of independence from your partner is just as crucial as having things in common – but there must also be a substantial degree of overlap when it comes to the way you want your lives to look in the future.

What we want in a relationship is dictated by both our goals for the future, and our values, beliefs and desires. When our innermost beliefs and values are challenged by our partner, it can lead to conflict and misunderstandings. And when we simply don't know or understand our partner's dreams and goals for the future, it can have similarly disastrous results.

One thing successful companies, businesses and individuals have in common is their use of vision statements. These statements essentially work as a guidepost, showing them the way towards a shared goal. And just like business owners and entrepreneurs, couples can also benefit from creating their own vision statement.

Creating a vision for your relationship – and putting it down on paper – is a helpful way to ensure both you and your partner are on the same track; to ensure your values are in alignment with one another's (more on this in Chapter Six) and ensure your lives are headed in the same direction.

Everyone enters a relationship with a preconceived idea about the way they want things to be. These ideas might stem from your parents' marriage, previous relationships, or even things we see on TV or social media. Far too often, couples fail to communicate these ideas with other, leading to irreparable rifts.

Co-creating a shared relationship vision helps you both get clear on exactly what is important to you, both in your relationship and in life as a whole. It helps outline the steps you must take in order to reach the life of your dreams – both as individuals and as a couple. Essentially, a relationship vision acts as a map to help you and your partner navigate the journey of your relationship and your shared lives.

How to Create a Relationship Vision

Step One: Take a blank piece of paper each and, separately, spend some time brainstorming about what constitutes your perfect relationship. For each element, write a short sentence in present tense, as though the things you envisage have imagined has already come into fruition. Your list might include things like "We share openly with each other," "We are doting parents," "We have a great sex life" or "We travel a lot." There is no right or wrong here; just use your imagination and write what feels good to you. Be sure to phrase each statement in a positive way. For example, rather than writing "We never fight," you could write "We discuss our differences in a calm and loving way."

As you compile your list, take into account every area of your life, including:

- Communication
- Your career
- Your home/life balance
- Sex and romance
- Your relationship with each other's family
- Parenting

- Leisure time
- Lifestyle
- Living arrangements

Consider elements such as how you handle conflict, how you relate to one another and how you make decisions.

For each statement, mark down whether it is simply a desirable aspect of your ideal relationship, or whether it is non-negotiable to you.

Once you have each written a minimum of six statements, take turns reading each sentence out loud to each other. Hold back any comments or judgements at this time. You will have a chance to speak in detail about each other's lists, but the goal for now is simply to listen and share.

Depending on how open you have been with your partner in the past, you may find this part of the exercise a challenge. But remember, the more transparent you and your partner are with each other, the stronger your relationship will be as a result.

Step Two: Now you have shared your ideal relationship traits with each other, it's time to compare lists. Go through item by item, and whenever you find a shared or similar statement, mark it with a tick.

Next, go through your partners list and look at the unticked items. If there are any statements that you agree with but did not put on your own list, add it now. You can then mark these with a tick.

Now take a look at the remaining items – the statements on each other's lists on which you cannot agree. Underline these statements.

Step Three: Taking all your shared statements, compile them into one list on a fresh piece of paper. This is now your relationship vision. Read it aloud to each other, taking turns to read a statement one at a time. Is there anything you feel is missing and needs to be added?

It is important to remember that this vision is not set in stone. As you grow as people and as a couple, your goals and values are likely to change somewhat and it is important to update your relationship vision to represent this. Put your list somewhere you will both see it regularly and make changes to it whenever you see fit.

Step Four: So what about those underlined statements on your lists; the relationship points that you and your partner could not agree on?

Of course, it would not be healthy do simply sweep these under the rug and pretend they don't exist. Nor should they be an automatic red flag for your relationship.

If you find yourself disagreeing with the majority of each other's statements, it could well be a sign that you and your partner are incompatible, and you should look closely at the values of both yourself and your partner to determine whether the relationship is worth persisting with. If you disagree with a number of each other's non-negotiable relationship aspects, it can be a big red flag in your relationship. (More on this in Chapter Six.)

But if you feel confident that you are with the right person, regardless of a few disagreements, you can view these statements as an opportunity for discussion and growth. We will be looking further at techniques for improving communication and discussion in Chapter Seven. Of course, this is also where seeking the help of a professional relationship counsellor can be of great value.

Exercises:

CHAPTER SIX: YOUR PERSONAL VALUES

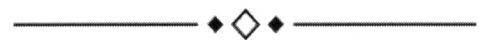

As we touched on in the previous chapter, one of the most important foundations on which to build and grow a partnership is the presence of shared personal values. In other words, you are you partner share the same fundamental beliefs about what is important in your lives and in the world in general.

When we first begin dating, these deeper values may be of secondary importance. Instead, we welcome the great time we have with a person, or how much fun they are to be around. But when you want your partner to be someone you can spend your life with, rather than just someone you have fun with now and then, personal values grow immensely in importance.

Our personal values are an intrinsic part of who we are. They constitute the things you consider important in your personal life, working life and the world in general. Values determine your priorities in life and can be used as signposts to determine whether or not your life is turning out the way you had hoped or planned.

When you are living a life in line with your personal values, you often feel as though you are "in the flow" – that things are inherently easy. Life feels positive and uplifting, and you often feel a deep sense of satisfaction as you go through your day. Conversely, when you are living out of harmony with your values, life can just feel "wrong." You may feel as though you are living the life chosen for you by someone else, or that you have somehow ended up in a life that is wildly different from the one you intended to live. Living outside of your values can be a source of deep unhappiness. It can also cause you to lose sight of your true self, and who you really are.

Hopefully the above highlights just how important values are, both to our sense of self, and to our relationship. But what exactly does it mean to share values with someone? In essence, it means you value the same things in life; that you have similar beliefs about what is important to you as an individual, as a couple and to life in general. For example, you may both share a belief in marriage and a traditional family setting; you may value honesty and openness, or freedom and spontaneity. Religious, spiritual and political beliefs can also come under the umbrella of personal values.

Identifying your Own Values

The first step when determining whether or not your partner shares your values is to get clear on exactly what's important to you. You may already have a clear idea of what your values are, but it's possible that you are yet to reach that point of clarity.

The following exercise will assist you in getting clear on just what is important to you. It will help you identifying your key values, within a relationship, as an individual and in the world at large. You will need something to write on, along with a quiet place in which you will not be interrupted. Be sure to answer each question as honestly as possible . Do not to censor yourself – just let the words come out without judgement. Allow your responses pour onto the paper without overthinking them. Your subconscious may bring up some answers that you were not expecting. If you find this is the case, be open to the process and what might reveal itself.

- *Step One: Identify the times in life when you felt the happiest*

  Think about instances in your personal life, family life and career when you felt completely filled with joy. What were you doing? Who were you with? Where were you? What other factors contributed to that feeling of utter happiness? Write down as much detail as you can about these times. Remember, it does not have to be something as huge as traveling the globe (although if that fills you with joy, great!). Maybe you felt the happiest when you were at home up on the sofa with your loved ones or pets. Write from the heart and find the things that made *you* happiest, not the things you believe society says *should* have made you the most joyful.

- *Step Two: Identify the times in life when you felt most fulfilled.*

  Again, try to find examples from all areas of your life; personal, family, social and work. Examine exactly what need or desire the experience filled, and why it was so important to you. In what way did the experience give meaning to your life?

- *Step Three: Identify the times in life when you felt the proudest.*

  Again considering all areas of your life, ask yourself exactly what it was about these moments that made you feel proud. Who were you with? Did you feel proud of yourself, of others, or both? In what way did the experience help give your life meaning?

- *Step Four: Identify times in which you felt bad.*

  In this step, we will use "bad" to mean any one of a number of negative emotions. Maybe acting in a particular way made you feel guilty, or frustrated or sad. Examine exactly what emotion the activity or event made you feel. Who were you with? Where were you? Exactly what was it about the event or activity that made you feel these negative emotions? Be as honest and open with yourself as you can.

- *Step Five: Identify things other people have done that you admire.*

  Here, consider times you have looked up to people, or been impressed by another's achievements and/or behavior. Clarify exactly what each person did and why it is something you aspire to do or be. Why is this important to you? Once again, be as specific and honest with yourself as possible, and remember to use your own instinct to answer the question. Do not simply include things you feel you *should* admire – all too often we conform ourselves to what we believe society is telling us to feel. Be conscious of falling into this trap.

- *Step Six: Identify things others did that you resented or did not approve of.*

  As with the previous step, the answer to this question can focus on any number of negative emotions, situations or behaviors. Perhaps the government did something that infuriated you, or a friend said something to upset you. Were you frustrated by a workmate's actions, or are there behaviors of society at large that you wish you could change? Again, be as clear and specific as you can. Write down details of the exact situation and who it was that made you feel the negative emotions. Where did the event or activity occur and exactly what was it about it that made you feel these negative emotions? Describe in detail how it made you feel. Be as honest and in depth as possible.

- *Step Seven: Identify your key values from the list below.*

  Now read through your answers for the first three questions. Can you see any patterns appearing?

  The following list contains a series of values that we adopt and live by in various areas of our lives. You will notice that several of these values are directly related to romantic relationships, such as marriage and family, while others are broader.

  Go through the list and circle or highlight those you feel resonate most with you, based on your answers to the above questions. Remember to trust your instinct – you may find yourself drawn to an answer you were not expecting.

Accountability

Accuracy

Accepting challenges

Achievement

Adventurousness

Ambition

Assertiveness

Balance

Belonging

Beauty

Boldness

Clarity

Class

Commitment

Community

Competition

Consistency

Contribution

Control

Courtesy

Creativity

Curiosity

Decisiveness

Development

Discipline

Diversity

Effectiveness

Empathy

Enthusiasm

Equality

Excellence

Excitement

Expression

Fairness

Faith

Family

Fitness

Friendship

Fun

Generosity

Goodness

Growth

Happiness

Harmony

Honesty

Honor

Humility

Improvement

Independence

Insightfulness

Intelligence

Intuition

Joy

Justice

Leadership

Level-headedness

Love

Loyalty

Making a difference

Marriage

Mastery

Maternalism

Obedience

Openness

Originality

Partnership

Passion

Paternalism

Patriotism

Perfection

Philanthropy

Positivity

Power

Preparedness

Quality

Reliability

Resourcefulness

Restraint

Rigor

Romance

Security

Self-control

Self-reliance

Serenity

Service

Simplicity

Speed

Spontaneity

Strength

Success

Stability

Spirituality

Teamwork

Thoughtfulness

Trust

Truth

Understanding

Uniqueness

Uninhibitedness

Unity

Victory

Vision

- *Step Eight: Create a list of your top five values*

  From the list of circled values, prioritize those you consider to be the five most important. This can be a difficult step as it requires you to look deep inside yourself. In searching for the answer to this question, think back to the answers you gave to the exercise in Chapter One in which we determined your un-purpose. Which of these values most closely align to this?

  When deciding which of these values are most important to you, it can be helpful to imagine yourself in different scenarios and determine which one resonates more strongly with you and your un-purpose. For example, if you are struggling to choose between the values of teamwork and success, you might ask yourself whether you would choose to be part of a close-knit sports team that is mediocre on the field or be at the top of your game in a solo sport such as running.

  Really take your time to identify your values. Doing so correctly may take days, or even weeks, but it is well worth the effort. Remember, these values are to become your guideposts as you live your life on un-purpose, so it is crucial to identify them correctly. Don't rush the process.

What did you learn from this process? Perhaps you already had a strong idea of what your personal values entailed. If so, did these questions bring up any unexpected answers?

Did the exercise help you gain clarity on exactly what is important to you as you go through life? Did it remind you of values that you had let fall to the wayside?

Sharing Your Values with Your Partner

In any relationship, the more values we share, the stronger our relationship is going to be. In Chapter Six we looked at a number of questions couples can ask each other to help better connect and begin to understand each other's values.

Once you have completed the above exercise and gained clarity on what's important to you, ask you partner to do the same. Allow them time and space to complete the exercise at their own pace; remember, sometimes answers to the above questions take many days to surface. Be patient and don't rush the process.

Once you have both completed the exercise, it's time to share your answers with each other.

What to Do When Your Values Don't Align

So you and your partner have shared your results of the values exercise. Likely you have learned a lot both about yourselves and each other and may have important additions to make to your relationship vision. (See Chapter Five.)

But what happens when you are your partner don't see eye to eye on a number of issues? Does that automatically spell the end for your relationship? Not necessarily.

While disagreements in certain areas – namely money, lifestyle, religion, politics and sex – can undoubtedly lead to challenges in a relationship, these disagreements don't necessarily mean a relationship is doomed.

Think back to the relationship vision exercise. What were the key aspects of the relationship that you deemed non-negotiable? While it is difficult to build a successful partnership whose views on these must-have items differs, variance in other areas can be a source of growth and understanding for both you and your partner.

So how do you go about successfully navigating a relationship when your views differ on a number of areas? It all comes down to respect and communication. Think of it this way; in even the strongest of relationships there will be issues on which partner disagree. This may be something as simple as what to eat for dinner, or something as critical as how to raise the children.

If you and your partner are having difficulties resolving differences in opinion, here are a few helpful steps to take:

Discuss the issue in detail.

While this may seem like an obvious first step, the keys here are openness and active listening. When your partner is explaining their thoughts on the matter at hand, be sure to pay close attention to what they are saying; don't just wait for your turn to speak. Allow your partner to make their point, and resist the urge to argue, or speak over them. When it is your turn to respond, do so without criticizing your partner's values, thoughts or beliefs. Express your views on the matter in a calm and clear manner and stick to talking about what it is you feel or believe, rather than attacking your partner's view.

It is possible that, through openly discussing the issue, you realize your values are not as out of alignment as you first believed. But even if this is not the case, openly discussing the matter will give you a better understand of where you partner stands; and will create firm footing for you to progress towards a compromise.

Try to understand where your partner is coming from.

Remember that often our beliefs are instilled in us very early on in life; we adopt values as a result of our parents, teachers or other caregivers. So when you and your partner are faced with a difference of opinion, endeavor to find out why they believe what they do. Is there something from their upbringing that has caused them to act, or believe, in the way they do? What kind of environment did they grow up in? What sort of family or friends do they have?

It can also help to examine your own values in the same way. Where do they come from? Are your beliefs truly your own or are they beliefs you have adopted that you have just never thought to question. By doing this, you may even find that you have outgrown your old beliefs or values.

Try to find common ground.

Even though you and your partner disagree on a particular issue, it is unlikely that you are unable to find any common ground. After all, if that was the case, you would likely not have been drawn to each other in the first place. When you are struggling to see eye to eye, take a step back and consider what fundamental beliefs you both share. For example, perhaps you both value openness and honesty. Or perhaps you both love the excitement and freedom of travel. Whatever your shared values, take a moment to identify, remember and appreciate them. How can these shared values be applied to the issue at hand?

Don't force your beliefs on your partner

While it can be frustrating when your partner views a key value in a different way to you, resist the temptation to thrust your views in their face. Forcing your beliefs on your partner will only increase the conflict. Depending on your partner's personality, they may also be inclined to crumble and accept your way of seeing things, in an attempt to relieve the conflict between you. While this may seem like an agreeable short-term solution, the reality is that this is far more likely to lead to deep-seated disagreements and unhappiness further down the track. Instead, acknowledge your differences and recognize them as an area in which you need to compromise and respect each other.

Acknowledge your boundaries.

This again comes back to your relationship vision and those elements you decided were non-negotiable. If, after careful and respectful discussion, you and your partner still have major issues you disagree on – such as whether or not to have children – it is important to consider whether or not the relationship is worth pursuing. Only you can truly know this, of course. But take the time to consider how your life would look if you gave up on one of your relationship must-haves. Is this a deal breaker for you? If so, it is best to confront this now. These major underlying issues are very unlikely to just go away; and sweeping them under the rug now will only lead to deeper and more heartbreaking problems in the future.

Exercises:

CHAPTER SEVEN: SECRETS TO IMPROVING YOUR COMMUNICATION

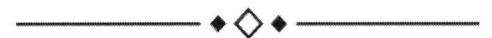

As we have seen to a degree already, no matter what the problem is in a relationship, good communication is the key to resolving the issues that can arise between you and your partner.

One of the biggest mistakes couple make is believing that any time they are talking, they are actually communicating. While talking, of course, is communication at a basic level, small talk about the weather, or work, or the kids does not address the deeper issues faced by many couples.

For many couples, the inability to communicate effectively is a problem they don't even know they have. Conversation may flow freely over the dinner table, and there may be little to no conflict, but nor is there anything meaningful discussion – discussion that goes to the heart of underlying problems within a relationship.

But learning to communicate on a deeper level is perhaps the most important thing you can do to improve the quality of your relationship. Improved communication leads to less misunderstandings and disagreements and allows you to resolve conflicts in a mature and respectful manner.

Let's take a look at some of the most important things to consider as you go about improving your communication skills:

Listen actively

So often when someone is speaking to us, our minds are actually losing focus – and this often happens without us being aware of it. Despite our best intentions, we tend to drift away from the present moment, away from what is being communicated, getting lost in our own thoughts.

Our ability to listen is also hampered by subconscious interpreting and agreeing or disagreeing. When someone is communicating with us, we filter the information through our own biases, drawing conclusions about the topic – or indeed, the speaker themselves – without really absorbing what they are saying. Next time you are listening to someone speak, try to catch yourself doing these things. After all, becoming aware you are doing something is the first step to changing it.

Active listening is perhaps the most important skill of all to develop when it comes to improving communication. All too often, when we are in a conversation with someone, we are not truly listening to what they are saying; instead, we are just waiting for our turn to speak. But when we actively listen to what is being said to us, it sends a powerful message to the speaker that what they are saying is worthwhile and valued. It makes it clear to our partner that their thoughts and opinions are important.

Active listening begins with being attentive. Make eye contact with the speaker and ensure you are in the present moment; not letting your mind drift into the past or future. Wait until your partner has finished speaking before you respond. If you are unclear about any elements of what they said, ask for clarification. This simple step goes a long way to showing that they have had your full attention.

Once your partner has finished and you have clarified anything you were uncertain about, respond to them by paraphrasing what they said. For example: "I understand you are angry that I haven't been spending enough time with you…" You can also use this time as an opportunity to show their concerns are recognized and valid, such as: "I know it must have been a surprise for you when I told you I wanted to quit my job…"

Another helpful technique to engage in active listening is drawing parallels to your own experiences. While of course, the aim here is not to make the issue "all about you," offering moments from your own life in which you felt the same, or similar, can go a long way towards showing your partner that you understand their side of the story.

Don't make assumptions.

In relationships, just as in many other areas of life, we as humans are prone to leaping to conclusions. We tell ourselves we know what a person in thinking, when in truth, we often have no idea – after all, how could we? None of us are mind readers.

Never assume you know what your partner is thinking; this can lead to conflict, misunderstandings and hurt. Rather than making assumptions, be open and willing to share, thus encouraging your partner to speak their mind.

Pay attention to body language and tone of voice.

While researchers disagree on exact numbers, most of us are in agreement that the majority of communication (some researchers claim up to 90%) is non-verbal. What this means is that the actual words we say are only a tiny part of the equation when it comes to communicating effectively. The rest comes down to tone and voice and body language. In other words, it's not necessarily *what* we say that matters, but rather *how* we say it.

Being aware of non-verbal signals is important when both listening and speaking. Non-verbal signals go a long way towards telling us whether the person we are speaking to is being truthful, if they are really listening, and if they care about what is being said. It tells us how they are feeling on a deeper level, often expressing far more than mere words can.

Paying attention to the way your partner is holding themselves physically can give you important clues as to how they are truly feeling. It is equally important that you pay attention to your own body language, to become aware of the signals you are sending to your partner when you are speaking.

Non-verbal communication serves several important roles:

1. *Repetition* – it can reinforce and compliment the message you are delivering through speech.
2. *Contradiction* – it can undermine the words you are saying; often a key indicator that you are not telling the truth.
3. *Substitution* – it can take the place of a verbal message. Our facial expressions provide an insight into how we are really feeling, communicating messages we are unable to verbalize. For example, looking into the eyes of someone can wordlessly communicate if they are scared, or bewildered. It can also impart positive feelings like love.
4. *Accenting* – non-verbal cues can highlight the importance of a verbal message. For example, pounding a fist against the table shows that your anger is particularly acute.

Here are some elements to take note of when becoming more aware of non-verbal communication:

– *Facial expressions*

The human face is capable of communicating countless emotions without a single word. It often offers far more insight into a person's true feelings than words can. In addition, facial expressions cross language and cultural barriers, meaning they are able to be understood by anyone, regardless of whether or not they share your native tongue.

– *Posture*

The way we hold ourselves when speaking is also a key indicator of how we truly feel about a matter. For example, folding your arms around your body indicates you are feeling defensive, afraid or closed off, while angling yourself towards a person indicates you are open to what they have to say.

– *Eye contact*

Making or breaking eye contact is often the element that determines whether or not a speaker is being truthful. If someone looks down while they are speaking to you, it can be a red flag that they are lying. Avoiding eye contact suggests you are either not interested in what your partner has to say, or else you are finding it difficult to say something, out of shame, embarrassment, or worry over how the other person will react.

– *Touch*

This element can be considered particular important when it comes to communicating with your spouse. Something as simple as a gentle hand on the arm can go a long way toward showing your partner you are connected and committed to working through issues as a team. Think about how different a conversation can feel if you are sitting side by side on the sofa, letting your knees rest against each other's, compared to sitting on opposite sides of the room with your arms folded against your chests. Though the content of the conversation may be the same, the former provides a much more welcoming environment for openness and connection.

But touch can also work the other way. Be aware of gestures that appear dominating or aggressive, such as a firm grip on your partner's arm.

– *Space*

The distance between two people who are conversing also goes a long way towards determining the atmosphere and hidden meaning of the discussion. Think back to the previous example of a couple sitting beside each other, compared to the couple sitting on opposite sides of the room. But just like touch, getting close to a person can indicate a desire for dominance – unwelcomingly invading a person's personal space can be construed as an act of aggression, regardless of how intimately you know each other.

– *Tone of Voice*

The way we say things often tells us a lot more about the meaning than the actual words. Pay attention to tone, inflection, pacing and volume of both your own words, and your partner's. Does your tone of voice indicate anger, frustration or sarcasm? Are you offering asides such as "yeah" or "I see" to indicate you are following what is being said?

Anticipate struggles and talk them through.

If you foresee trouble on the horizon, be open with your partner about it. For example, you may have a difficult few weeks of work coming up, or a difficult family gathering. Being open with your partner about potential struggles and letting them know what to expect helps them understand that your difficult behavior is not about them. It also gives them a chance to support you however they can.

Show gratitude

In relationships, like many other areas of life, when we are thankful for something, we create space to bring more of the good stuff into our lives. Even if you and your partner are facing major challenges, take a moment to think about something they have done – or some part of who they are – that you are truly grateful for. Maybe they made you your favorite dinner when you came home from work or put the kids to bed so you could have a night off, or perhaps they are always a good listener. It doesn't matter how big or small it is, be sure to acknowledge the behaviors and actions you appreciate. Once you have identified the thing you are grateful for, tell them. Thanking your partner for who they are and what they have done sends a powerful signal that you value them, regardless of whatever challenges you are currently facing.

Believe that things can change.

When you are facing difficulties in your relationship, it can be all too easy to believe that you will be stuck in this cycle of conflict forever. But that is simply not the case. You have already given a signal to yourself that you want change – you did that when you first picked up this book. Improving your communication skills is an important next step in working through your troubles, no matter how entrenched and unfixable they may feel. Believing that change is possible is the first step to making it so.

Exploring Your Relationship Together

In Chapter Four: Getting to Know Your Partner, we looked at a number of questions you and your spouse can ask each other to learn new things about what makes you both tick. In this chapter, as we continue to develop and build our communication skills, we will look at a number of deeper questions, specifically relating to your relationship.

These questions are a helpful way of identifying snags or ruts in your relationship – and they also serve to remind you why you fell in love with your spouse in the first place. Often, there are many things in our relationships that we take for granted; such as the fact that our partner makes us feel safe, or we have someone to chat to about our day when we get home. These questions will help shine a light on these important relationship elements.

But perhaps most importantly, these questions can be a less confronting way of raising issues that we struggle to confront or articulate, such as trust, or sexual problems. As always, when asking each other these questions, take time to listen to your partner's responses in a respectful and active way, adopting the methods of positive communication we have discussed in this chapter.

Relationship Questions

What is your favorite memory of our time together?

What is your favorite sexual memory of you and me?

When did you last think of me in a positive way?

What is one thing I do for you that you enjoy?

Which of my physical features do you like best?

When did you know you wanted to be in a relationship with me?

Of the things I do in bed, which do you enjoy the most?

What do you think is the biggest challenge in our relationship?

Do you believe I love you?

What could I do to make you trust me even more?

Is there a question you have always wanted to ask me but have never found the courage?

What makes me different to other partners you have had in the past?

Exercises:

CHAPTER EIGHT: HOW TO MASTER AND CONTROL THE EMOTIONS

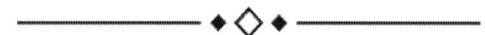

L et's take a step back now and consider the management of our own emotions. Often, when we find ourselves in a place of conflict with our partner, we act rashly, saying things we do not mean. This can lead to deep hurt, making issues harder to resolve.

While some level of conflict is inevitable in any relationship – even the most successful ones – losing your temper and acting rashly is not. When we learn to master and control our emotions, it puts us in a far better place to maturely communicate with our loved ones and resolve the issues that arise.

While this may sound easier said than done, the reality is, we do not need to be slaves to our emotions. After all, our emotions do not make us. They are simply passing thoughts – thoughts we can control.

There are many techniques we can adopt to better control our emotions. Let's take a look:

Develop Your Emotional Intelligence

The first step in controlling our emotions is learning to better understand them. Begin to see your feelings as separate from your core being. Your emotions do not define you; they change on a regular basis, so how can they? When you feel a particular emotion arise, take a moment to observe it. Do not try to change it, or make it go away. Simply recognize what it is you are feeling. Is it a positive or negative feeling? Can you be more specific? Perhaps it's disappointment, or embarrassment, or betrayal. Are you feeling bitter, or frustrated or horrified. Maybe you're feeling joy, or excitement or exhilaration. Being able to identify categorize your feelings in this way is the first step in releasing the control they have over you.

Once you have identified exactly what it is you are feeling, take a moment to observe what that emotion is doing to your body. Do you feel butterflies in your stomach, or is your heart pounding? Are your muscles feeling tenser than usual? If so, where? Acknowledge that even though the emotion may have a profound effect on your physical body, it is *not* your body. In other words, recognize that, even though you may be feeling a particular emotion very intensely, this emotion does not define you as a person. It is simply something that will pass.

Acknowledge the role your emotions play in supporting you

As we touched on above, mastering your emotions is not about ignoring the way you are feeling, or putting up a wall against negative feelings. Instead, it is about acknowledging them as an important part of yourself. Begin to see your emotions as a helpful thing; guideposts that help determine whether or not you are on the correct path in life. Instead of criticizing yourself for feeling a certain way, dig deeper into the way you are feeling, to determine the message that comes with this emotion. To do this, ask yourself the following questions:

- What is this particular emotion offering me in this moment?
- How does this emotion serve me?
- What action can I take to make this situation or emotion better?
- What beliefs do I need to have to get the outcome I desire?
- What is it that I truly desire?
- How can I learn from this experience to improve my emotional control in the future? What can I do better?

Above all, don't attempt to negate your emotions, or convince yourself they are wrong. Nothing you feel is "wrong" – and trying to convince yourself otherwise is the best way to block communication from your inner self and intuition.

Deep Breathing

Deep breathing has a wide range of both physical and mental benefits. It allows us to reduce stress, anxiety and tension, along with slowing the heart rate and lowering the blood pressure. As a result, it becomes a powerful tool to be utilized when our emotions are threatening to overwhelm us. The simple action of inhaling for five counts and exhaling for five counts, while focusing on the breath allows the mind to still, momentarily taking us away from the troublesome emotion. Often this moment is enough to give us a new perspective on the situation and view the circumstances more clearly and calmly.

Develop Your Communication

As we know from Chapter Seven, good communication is one of the key elements of a successful relationship. And when we improve our communication, we also improve our ability to handle our emotions. When we are able to speak more openly with our partner, we give ourselves the opportunity to share our needs and desires. Often the simple act of talking about an emotion is enough to take away its destructive power.

Have New Experiences.

Another useful technique for developing greater control over our emotions is to engage in new experiences. This can be anything from trying new foods, traveling to new places, learning a new language or watching a new film. When we engage in new activities, we are forcing our brain to form new concepts, and to view old ideas in new ways; essentially broadening our horizon. When we do this, we are increasing the brain's capacity to deal with our emotions, in a new and more positive way.

Focus on the Positives

As we know, focusing on the positives and being grateful for what we have is a surefire way to bring more good into our lives. Conversely, when we focus on the negatives, we are unconsciously drawing more negativity into our lives. Learning to master our emotions is no different. Next time you feel your emotions running away with you, think back to a time when you experienced this same feeling and were able to successfully control it. The fact that you did this in the past is a timely reminder that you are able to do it again. You may even like to keep a physical record of times in which you managed your emotions in a positive way. The next time you begin to feel out of control, you can look back on this record and see what you are truly capable of.

Exercises:

CHAPTER NINE: RESOLVING
FINANCIAL CONFLICT

It's likely that you and your partner have had at least one disagreement over money over the course of your relationship. After all, conflicts over financial matters are among the leading causes of divorce and relationship breakups. This is largely due to the powerful emotions that are often tied to our financial state. Thanks to societal pressures, we often equate our earning capacity with our self-worth, making finances a difficult subject for many people to broach.

So how should you go about navigating this particular minefield? As we have discussed already in this book, the crucial first step in resolving disagreements is up front communication. (If you haven't read Chapter Seven: Secrets to Improving Your Communication already, go back and do so now.) This step is just important when discussing financial issues as it is in any other disagreement.

When facing conflict around financial issues, whether that be overspending, disagreements on purchasing decisions or anything else connected to your economic well-being, openness and honesty is the key. Using the active listening techniques discussed in Chapter Seven, take time to share your feelings on the issue with your partner, being as honest and open as possible. Being able to see your partner's point of view on the issue will form the groundwork for compromise and healthy resolution of the issue at hand.

Let's now take a look at some specifics techniques that can be used when dealing with financial conflict.

Examine the root cause of your feelings around money.

As touched on above, for many people, conflict around money stems from a fear of it. Does talking about money bring up negative feelings for you? Do you have any idea why that might be? Often, our attitude around money is the direct result of our past; our beliefs stemming from our parents, or our early economic circumstances.

If you and your partner are experiencing conflict around money, it can be helpful to first examine your own beliefs around this subject. Many of us, often unconsciously, have limiting beliefs when it comes to our finances. Often these beliefs come as a result of the things we heard about money at a young age. Think back to your childhood and what your parents or caregivers told you about money. Did you hear phrases like "Money doesn't grow on trees" or "Money is the root of all evil?" If you grew up repeatedly hearing this, it can lead you to believe that we must struggle for money, or that being rich somehow equates to being bad. Conversely, if you grew up in a household in which you were never lacking, with caregivers who held beliefs such as "There is enough money for everyone who is willing to earn it" you are far more likely to view your financial situation from a place of abundance – and your bank balance will reflect this. Often, it is this difference in mindset that makes the difference between the wealthy and the poor.

Fully understand what is causing your attitude towards money – along with your partner's attitude – will help you give you both a better understanding about where the conflict stems from. For example, if you believe that money is difficult to come by and must be dutifully tucked away, while your partner believes in abundance and free spending, it will make the root of any misunderstanding clearer. It doesn't matter if the attitudes you uncover are positive or negative; for now, the only goal is understanding.

Once you are able to move past your hang-ups over money, you will be much better placed to make more positive and informed financial decisions – and discuss the issues more openly and calmly.

Resolving limiting beliefs about money

While the resolution of negative beliefs is largely outside the scope of this book, the key thing to take away here is to understand that all negative beliefs can be changed. Remember that a belief is just that; your own unique way of viewing the world – not an ingrained truth. If you have uncovered your own limiting beliefs around money, acknowledge that recognizing these beliefs is an important first step. It can be useful to write these beliefs down on a piece of paper. From here, consider what you would like to replace your limiting belief with. For example, if you believe "It's not fair to be rich when so many others are poor", consider replacing this with a more positive belief such as "I can help people more easily when I have more money." Continue to repeat your new beliefs to yourself over and over until they begin to take root.

See yourself and your partner as a team

This is a key element of a successful relationship, and among the most important aspects when it comes to creating a comfortable dialogue around money. Remember that a relationship is not about winning or losing; rather it is about uniting with your partner and facing the world together. When you view yourselves in this way, you strengthen your relationship in all areas, including the financial arena.

Create separate budgets for personal spending

Often, conflict around money arises when one partner does not approve of the other's spending habits. This can lead to one partner trying to hide their purchases from the other, resulting in arguments when the clandestine purchases are discovered.

These days, it is not unusual for couples to have individual bank accounts, and this can help eradicate the need for hiding guilt purchases. But even if you and your partner share an account, the problem can be avoided by creating individual budgets. Each week, or month, allocate funds to both a shared, or family account, along with individual funds that can be spent by each partner as they wish. Once this money has been divided, it is up to each individual to spend their money as they see fit, and they should be able to do so without fear of being reprimanding from their partner.

Ensure your relationship vision and values encompass finance

When you and your partner have guiding principles to operate by, it makes navigating conflict easier. And, needless to say, outlining these principles is much simpler, and more productive outside of a stressful, conflict-fueled argument. Through the relationship vision exercise (Chapter Five) and/or the exercises in identifying your values (Chapter Six) make sure you and your partner understand what is important to you when it comes to finances. Is it important to you to save for a deposit on a house, or do you value freedom and travel, for example? Remember, there is no right or wrong answer here, what's important is that you communicate your desires, believes and values to your partner and listen actively as they communicate their own.

Consult a financial advisor

While a relationship counselor is a fantastic person to turn to in order to navigate the marital difficulties, when conflict arises over finances, a financial advisor or accountant can also be a great help. Often, seeking help from a professional will help set you on the right path, and remove the stress that arises from managing your own finances.

A financial advisor can help you plan for the future, and ensure your personal finances are on the right track. Perhaps most importantly, a professional will help you make informed, level-headed decisions about your financial future, rather than relying on the emotions that can take over in the heat of a conflict. When you are your partner are forced to confront your financial issues in the presence of a professional third party, it can lead you to reconsider the situation in a more objective and balanced way.

Make a financial plan

Whether or not you choose to enlist the help of a financial advisor, or go it alone, putting time into creating a financial plan can take much of the stress out of managing your personal economic situation. When your shared – and personal goals – are clearly laid out, the result is less conflict and less arguments.

A financial plan is of particular importance if you and your partner are newly married, expecting a child or buying a property. It can also be a major help in easing conflict and improving your financial outlook.

Needless to say, a financial plan should be something that both you and your partner create together. Although the detailed creation of a financial plan is outside the scope of this book (you will find endless information about how to do this online) here are some steps to consider when creating your plan, and in particular, how financial planning directly relates to the health of your relationship.

- *Begin with where you are*

   The first step to improving your financial situation is to take a close look at where you are now. Look at your accounts, debts, savings and investments in close detail, ensuring you have accurate figures for all of the above. (If this elicits negative feelings for you, go back to the exercise above to uncover and remove any damaging or limiting beliefs you may have about money.)

- *Analyze your spending*

   Once you have a figure, think carefully about your spending habits. Now is not the time to be judgmental towards your partner; it is simply a time to be open with one another about your needs and desires. What do you need to spend money on each week that is non-negotiable? And what are some of your most important wants? Again, now is not the time to be critical of your partner if your desires seem to be out of line with each other's. It is simply a time to get everything out on the table and be as transparent as possible.

- *Consider what's important to you*

Now take time to consider what is important to you both in life; in other words, what you want to spend your money on. Remember not to censor yourself; ensure that you are considering things that you feel are important, not what society – or you partner – tells you you *should* think are important. If you value going out and having a good time over buying a house, that's fine; the key here is to be open and honest. When considering what's important to you, think back to your relationship vision. What elements of your dream life particularly pertain to your financial well-being? Above all, remember that this is a partnership – you must take into account not only your own wishes and desires, but also those of your partner. Are there areas in which your values are out of alignment with each other? In all likelihood, it's from here that the conflict arose in the first place. Is there a compromise you can reach in order to move forward?

Exercises:

CHAPTER TEN: SEXUAL CONNECTION
– HOW TO CREATE MORE INTIMACY

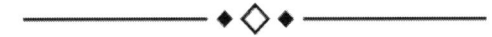

For many couples, issues arising in the bedroom can lead to deeper problems within the relationship. If you and your partner struggle to be sexually intimate, these problems can spill over into other areas of your life, causing a breakdown in connection at all levels.

While of course there are no set guidelines as to how often you and your partner should be having sex – some couples happily go months or even years without while others require it every day – it is important to address any issues surrounding sexual intimacy as early as possible.

Like many things in life, it is the quality of your sexual connection that matters, not how often you engage in intercourse. Employing some of the techniques below can assist you in creating a deeper connection with your partner – both physical and emotionally – leading to a better sex life, and a deeper connection on all levels.

Maintain physical contact and affection

Maintaining physical contact with your partner throughout the day is a key way to ensure the spark remains alive. This can be as simple as a quick kiss, a gentle hand on the back, or a hug. It's the simple act of making contact that shows your partner you love them and find them attractive.

Educate yourself

In today's information age, there is no shortage of material both on and offline covering just about every sexual issue you can think of. Find some resources that apply to your particular situation, sharing them with your partner. While it's great to be able to discuss this openly, many couples find this difficult to do. Alternatively, consider highlighting or underlining passages you find relevant, then sharing the reference with your partner. This can be an important first step in opening up dialogue around your sex life.

If openly discussing your sex life with your partner is a challenge for you, it can be helpful to consider why. Is it a matter of not trusting your partner enough, or has your upbringing lead you to believe that sexuality is not something that should be discussed openly? Whatever the reason, identifying the reason behind your reluctance can be an important first step to overcoming it.

Make time for sex

When the busyness of life overwhelms us, our sex lives often get neglected. And while it may sound unromantic, scheduling time for sex ensures it does not slip off the radar. This is particularly important if you have children who take up the majority of your time, or if you are getting older, when your sexual responses typically slow down and being intimate with your partner may require more time.

Discuss your sexual fantasies

If you and your partner are able to talk openly about sex, it does not just mean you'll be more fulfilled in the bedroom. It means you are deeply connected and much more able to be open with each other in every aspect of your lives. After all, our sexual fantasies are one of the most personal aspects of ourselves, and when we trust someone enough to share them, it lets them know we have the utmost faith in them. Talking openly with your partner about your sexual fantasies lays the groundwork for deeper trust and openness, not to mention a more exciting sex life.

Communicate during sex

This does not necessarily mean engaging in dirty talk – although if that's your thing, great. Rather, it's about improving your levels of intimacy by giving your partner cues to make sex more pleasurable for both of you. These could be verbal cues, or simple instructions, or even just the act of guiding your partner's hands. As close as you are, you cannot expect your partner to read your mind – and letting your partner know exactly what turns you on will make the experience more memorable for both of you.

Relax

Particularly if you and your partner have been having issues in the bedroom, sex can become a stressful event. To relieve anxiety, be sure to engage a relaxing activity beforehand. This could include going out for dinner, doing yoga, meditation or deep breathing exercises, or even just giving each other a back rub. The activity itself it not important; it's all about ensuring that when you make it to bed, you have no anxiety or concerns about what is about to happen.

Practice the Sensate Focus Technique.

A technique widely used by sex therapists, Sensate Focus is used to help increase people's enjoyment of sex, while deepening their connection to their partner. It operates on the basis of "mindful sex," helping people get out of their heads in order to fully enjoy their body. As much of the technique actually prohibits the touching of the breasts and genitals, Sensate Focus is far more about awakening one's sensuality, rather than their sexuality – in turn, deepening their connection to both their own body, and their partner.

To begin, decide which of you will be the "toucher" and who will be the "receiver." Take a shower beforehand and remove your clothes, along with any watches or jewelry. Find a time and place where you will not be interrupted. If you have been designated the "receiver" find a position in which you can lie down comfortably. If you are the "toucher," spend at least fifteen minutes exploring your partner's body, avoiding the genitals and breasts. Pay attention to how the texture of his or her skin changes in different parts of the body. Compare the skin on the back of the arm, for example, to the skin on the cheek. Now, vary the tempo and pressure of your touch. How does this change your experience? Also try touching with different parts of your hand. Use one or two fingers for a while, then change to your palm, or the back of your hand. How does this change the experience? Note that the point here is not to arouse yourself or your partner, or to touch them in a way you think they will enjoy. It is simply an exercise in mindfulness and connecting with your own body, and that of your partner's.

Now change roles. As the "receiver," pay attention to the way each movement feels on your skin. How do the sensations change when your partner uses different speeds, or different parts of his/her hands to touch you? You may like to continue with this first step for several days, before moving on to the next part.

Step two involves the same mindfulness technique, this time allowing the touching of the breasts and genitals. Despite this, the aim is still mindfulness and awareness, rather than pleasure. As you implement this second step, you may find yourself instinctively drawn towards sexual touching. If that happens, slow down and return to the techniques used in step one; namely, focusing on the textures of your partner's body, and the different qualities of your touch. Don't focus on the touching of genitals – remember here the idea is not sexual contact, just a broader exploration.

At this point in the exercise you may choose to implement the "hand-riding technique" in which the receiver covers the toucher's hand with their own as he or she continues to explore their body. The aim here is not for the receiver to outwardly guide the toucher to where they want to be touched, but rather to impart any subtle non-verbal cues, such as where a heavier touch is welcome, or areas which are less or more sensitive. It's important to note here that the toucher should not interpret these cues as criticism, but rather as suggestions.

It is particularly important in this step to refrain from kissing, as this can lead into automatic sexual touching and responses, which is not the aim of this exercise. Often, kissing is a part of the old, routine sexual habits that the Sensate Focus technique aims to break.

Despite the fact that the goal here is not sexual touching, if the receiver finds themselves brought to orgasm, just let it happen; but do not aim for this outcome.

Like step one, you may wish to continue with this step for several days before moving on to the next one.

Step three removes the roles of "toucher" and "receiver" to allow for mutual sensual touching. The same rules apply as for step two – you may touch any area of your partner's body, though the goal is sensual exploration, rather than giving or receiving sexual pleasure. Continue to refrain from kissing.

If the routine nature of your sex life is something you are trying to break, consider doing this step in a location other than your bed, such as the shower, or living room, if you live alone.

Step four progresses to the act of sensual – not sexual – intercourse. Just as you did in step three, take time to enjoy the textures and shapes of each other's bodies, without having any particular goal in mind. From here, move to a position in which intercourse is physically possible. If you don't wish to engage in intercourse at this time, that's absolutely fine; simply continue with the sensual exploration of each other's bodies. But if you do wish to progress, be sure to do so in a slow and mindful way, taking note of the physical sensations and ensuring you remain in your body, not allowing your mind to drift, or to engage in sexual fantasies. Keep your focus on the sensations throughout, remembering that the goal here is simply to be present and mindful, not necessarily to reach orgasm.

The Sensate Focus technique is a method you can return to from time to time in order to break up any monotony in your sex life.

Exercises:

CHAPTER ELEVEN: REBUILDING TRUST IN YOUR RELATIONSHIP AFTER IT'S BEEN BROKEN

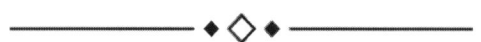

T rust is perhaps the most important element in a successful, happy and long-lasting relationship. Being able to trust our partner gives us an inherent sense of safety, and makes us comfortable being open and honest and revealing our true selves.

Trust can be broken by a number of things, such as infidelity, broken promises, or untruths. But if these things happen in your relationship, does it necessarily mean the end?

If you and your partner are truly committed to rebuilding your broken relationship, it can be done. Acknowledge that, if trust has been lost, the journey back can be a long one – but it is possible. It requires both parties to commit to reconnecting with each other and picking up the pieces of their relationship.

Psychologists agree there are five main areas which need to be addressed in order to rebuild broken trust. Let's take a look:

1. *Fully understand the situation*

    If you are the one who was betrayed, in order to re-establish trust in your partner, it is important that you first understand the exact situation that led to the trust being broken. What happened, when and where? What were the circumstances? Why do you think this happened? The aim here is not to make judgements, simply to view the situation from an objective, facts-based point of view.

If you are the partner who did the betraying, your duty here is to be as open and honest as possible, providing your partner with answers to all their questions.

2. *Letting go of your anger*

While this can certainly be easier said than done, it is important to take note of the effect anger can have on both your mental and physical well-being. Prolonged anger can lead to increased anxiety, high blood pressure and frequent headaches, as well as poor sleep, diminished appetite and mental stress.

To let go of the anger you are holding inside, you must first become fully aware of it. What emotions might you have bottled up, or refused to confront? What was the exact effect of your partner's betrayal? Did it trigger feelings of abandonment, or lack of self-worth? Did you feel as though you were made a fool or? Becoming fully aware of these feelings is an important step in releasing them. Now communicate these feelings to your partner, in a calm and rational manner.

This is also a chance for the partner who did the betraying to share their feelings. Likely, their poor behavior was triggered by negative emotions or beliefs, and they may be carrying around a similar amount of anger. It is just as crucial for the offender to identify their emotions, in order to release them, and prevent any further breaches of trust.

3. *Make your partner aware of your commitment*

When trust is broken, it can lead both the betrayer and betrayed to question their partner's commitment to rebuilding the relationship. If you have been betrayed, you may question whether your partner was committed to you in the first place, and if you were the offending party, you may consider whether your actions were too grievous for your partner to come back from.

But if there is to be a true rebuilding of trust, it is crucial that both parties reaffirm their commitment to each other. This is a chance for the betrayer to convey their regret or remorse, along with any other feelings they may be experiencing, such as frustration. And it is an opportunity for the betrayed to be open about their hurt. As you share your feelings with each other, try to do so from a place of empathy. Consider how your partner is feeling in this moment and do your best to support them.

From here, both parties must articulate what they need from the relationship in order to move forward. Do this in a calm and respectful manner, using non-blaming language such as "I need to feel loved," rather than "You made me feel unloved." Once you reach this step, the time for blaming is behind you, and it's important these statements reflect that.

4. ***Decide to forgive – or allow yourself to be forgiven.***

We talked in length about forgiving your partner in Chapter Three, so if you haven't done so already, go back and read this now. Remember that a big part of forgiveness is actively deciding to do so; choosing to no longer wish ill luck upon your partner who has betrayed you.

Conversely, if you are the one who has committed the offense, you may find it a challenge to allow yourself to be forgiven; in other words, you may find it difficult to forgive yourself for your actions. Because, while forgiving others can be a challenge, forgiving ourselves, particularly when we have committed an offense that has hurt our partner or put our relationship in jeopardy, can be much more difficult. Thanks to our inner critic – that negative voice we all have inside our head criticizing us and pointing out our failures– we have the tendency to replay negative events over and over. This causes us to dwell on our mistakes and punish ourselves far more harshly than we likely would if another person behaved in the same manner.

Forgiving ourselves requires many of the same skills as forgiving others; specifically, compassion, kindness and understanding, but it can be much more difficult to give these things to ourselves than to offer them to others. But if you and your partner are to rebuild trust and move on from the past, forgiving yourself is a crucial part. This is for a number of reasons, including:

- *The need for release.* When we are able to forgive ourselves, we release the physical tension we have been carrying inside our bodies; tension that, just like prolonged anger, can cause stress that leads to many physical and mental ailments.

- *It increases our capacity to forgive others.* We are unable to give away that which we don't have. If we are unable to forgive ourselves for our mistakes, it becomes much harder to forgive others. Think of the long lasting effect this can have on your relationship. How can you move forward if you are in a place where you would be unable to forgive your partner for any mistakes?

- *Forgiveness allows us to grow.* When we forgive ourselves and learn to move past our mistakes, we can reframe the past and learn from it instead of punishing ourselves on repeat. Our mistakes then become a source of growth that strengthen your relationship rather than destroying it.

If you find it particularly difficult to forgive yourself, you may like to consider the following steps:

- *Acknowledge and accept your emotions.* The first step in moving past our mistakes is acknowledging our emotions, as we discussed in Step Two. Take time to recognize exactly what it is you are feeling. Let your emotions rise to the surface, however painful they are, and give them a name. Are you disappointed in yourself? Angry? Frustrated? By acknowledging exactly what it is we are feeling, we have a firm starting point to forgive ourselves and repair our relationship with both our partner and ourselves.

- *Acknowledge the lesson at hand.* Any failures in life can be viewed as opportunities to learn. So too can situations in which you feel the need for self-forgiveness. In Step Two, you acknowledged the facts of your mistake and discussed it openly with your partner – this may have been difficult, but it was likely also quite therapeutic. Now consider what you can take from the situation? Perhaps it led you to recognize your need for more freedom within your relationship, or a deep-seated fear of being abandoned. How will understanding these things help you move forward in your relationship and develop as a person?

– *Connect with Your Inner Critic.* We mentioned our inner critic in the section above – it is that voice inside our head that is constantly criticizing us and making us question our abilities. Not only can this inner critic cause us to constantly doubt ourselves, but it is also the voice inside us that tells us we do not deserve to be forgiven. All too often, we attempt to silence our inner critic by attempting to ignore it, believing this is the only way to move past its destructive words. But connecting and conversing with this negative voice can actually be far more helpful. Begin to become aware of the thoughts that arise as your inner critic begins to speak. Can you identify the ways in which you are self-sabotaging your happiness and chance for forgiveness? For each comment that your inner critic makes, do your best to analyze it in an objective way. How true is this observation? For example, if your inner voice tells you "You've ruined your marriage and you'll never find happiness again," is this necessarily true? It may feel like it at times, but if you examine the situation from a more objective, level-headed viewpoint, you will see that it is in fact a lie. You and your partner are working to repair your broken relationship, and when you do so, it will lead you to happiness again.

For each self-destructive thought, try and replace it with a more compassionate and constructive response. For the above example, you may replace the above statement with "We are rebuilding our marriage and finding happiness along the way."

• *Give yourself time.*

It may be that you are simply not ready process the necessary emotions right now. Perhaps the negative emotions your mistake has aroused are threatening to overwhelm you and you don't feel as though you have the strength to work through your pain. If you find yourself in this position, first of all take a moment to accept that this is all right. Don't use the situation as yet another excuse to punish yourself, or convince yourself the relationship is over. Acknowledge that you made a mistake and will work through it in the near future when you are in a better frame of mind. Then, to stop yourself from dwelling on the negativity, and to stop it roiling away inside you, imagine removing the negative emotions from your body and locking them in a box.

Now picture yourself putting the box away somewhere safe. Give yourself permission to leave the box and the feelings within it to one side for now, in the knowledge that you will return to it when you feel you are ready.

– *Avoid dwelling on the past.* As we now know, a big part of forgiveness is consciously choosing to do so. When forgiving others, we choose to no longer wish them ill will and make the shift to a place of compassion and kindness. Similarly, when we are forgiving ourselves, we need to make a conscious decision to no longer beat ourselves up over our offence. If you continue to dwell on your mistakes, it can have as negative effect on your relationship as if your partner is the one to dwell on the past.

But not dwelling on the past is certainly easier said than done. As humans, we have a tendency to focus on our errors and can torture ourselves by replaying our mistakes over and over in our heads. This is especially true if our mistakes have put our marriage or relationship in jeopardy, or caused great harm to the one we love.

To stop yourself from constantly replaying the mistake in your head, it is first important to recognize you are doing it. Often these thoughts and negative experiences churn through our thoughts so automatically we are not aware of them, just of the negative feelings they evoke. When you catch yourself thinking of the past, stop and take note of it. Acknowledge exactly what thoughts are in your head and how they are making you feel. Now, instead of allowing yourself to continue to dwell on the experience, replace it with a positive action. This could be as simple as taking five long, deep breaths, going for a walk, or a favorite hobby, such as playing a musical instrument. Whatever the action is doesn't matter – the goal is to interrupt the negative thought pattern and replace it with something more positive and productive.

Once you have chosen to forgive yourself/your partner, this is where the work of rebuilding the relationship truly begins. As always, honesty and openness are the keys here, along with a number of other points to keep in mind:

If you are the offending party:

- It is not enough to simply tell your partner your behavior has changed. You need to actively show them. Embody the promises you made to yourself and your partner when you decided to move past the mistakes and rebuild your relationship.
- Consistently take responsibility for your actions. This means, not only the poor behavior that led the breakdown of your marriage in the first place, but all your actions moving forward.

If you are the party that was betrayed:

- Continuously work on understand what went wrong in your relationship. While this should not excuse your partner's behavior in any way, acknowledge that there may be areas of your own behavior that could be improved.
- Once you have made the decision to forgive your partner, engage in positive reinforcement to show them you appreciate the efforts they are making in improving their ways. Offer compliments when you can and, support them in their attempts to become a better person.
- Acknowledge that you always have the option of ending the relationship, even after you and your partner have completed the above steps. If you truly find it impossible to move past your partner's transgression, be honest about it. Carrying on with a relationship in which you are no longer invested will only lead to long-term tension and unhappiness for both of you.

When facing the challenge of rebuilding trust, it can be helpful to keep sight of the bigger picture. Remember why you fell in love in the first place, and focus on the goal of a renewed and long-lasting relationship, in which trust is paramount and central.

CHAPTER TWELVE: DISAGREEMENTS ABOUT PARENTING

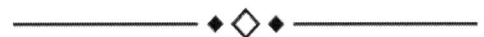

These days, unlike the past, it is not necessarily expected that couple will settle down and have children. As a result, most couples have a discussion about becoming parents before they make any long-lasting commitments to each other. But very few people sit down with their partner to discuss *how* they will raise their children. Often, this is simply because we have put little thought into the issues ourselves. Many of us just tell ourselves we will raise our children in much the same manner as we ourselves were raised. Needless to say, this can lead to a number of disagreements with your partner – particularly if they were raised in a very different manner to yourself.

The result is a clash in parenting styles, leading to tension in a marriage and confusion for the child or children. Often, the result of such clashes is for one parent to be seen as the "strict one," while the other is more lenient. The strict parent can get frustrated when their partner is too lenient, while the lenient partner can object to their spouse's hard-handed approach. As a result, both parties tend to amplify their behavior, with the strict parent becoming the stricter and the lenient parent relaxing their ways even further.

Needless to say, such conflict can be damaging not only for your relationship, but for your children as well. So what are some ways you can go about resolving disagreements that arise regarding parenting?

Communication is the key

You've heard it said many times already in this book, but it is worth saying again; the first step to resolving friction in your relationship is open and honest communication. While it is of course ideal to have discussed your parenting approaches with your partner before you have children, it is never too late to begin. Start by telling your partner exactly what style of parenting you grew up with, and how it affects your approach to your own children. Do you want to raise your children the same way that you were raised? Why or why not? Discuss issues with your partner such as what you both believe are effective disciplining techniques, as well as more specific topics such as appropriate bedtimes and household responsibilities. More likely than not, there will be areas you disagree on, making it necessary to compromise.

Come up with rules together

In the same way that you and your partner wrote down a list of your ideal relationship qualities when you completed the relationship vision exercise, take some time to write down a list of house rules, as relating to your children. The list can include items such as children's' bedtimes, allowances, permitted use of electronics and homework requirements. As you create this list, ensure the two of you are sharing the responsibility; don't let the "strict" parent automatically take the reins. In order for this to work, it must be a joint venture, just like the relationship vision.

Come up with consequences together

For each rule you determine, come up with set consequences that will happen if your children break one of the rules. Write these down. Once you have created the list of both rules and consequences, share them as a family. This will help children become clearer on what is required of them, and will ensure you and your partner don't come to any disagreements on punishments should the need arise.

Support each other in front of the children

Division and conflict comes when your children begin to recognise the "strict" parent and "lenient" parent. Remove this divide by ensuring that you and your partner remain on the same page in front of your children. When one partner makes a declaration in front of the kids, such as reprimanding them for bed language, or coming home later, it is crucial that the other partner backs him or her up. Failure to do so only heightens the divide between the "strict" and "lenient" parent, leading the children to test the boundaries of their lenient parent and increasing the conflict between you and your partner.

Exercises:

CHAPTER THIRTEEN: COUPLES AND SPIRITUALITY

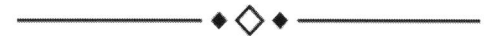

Along with finance, sex and parenting, another key issue that arises in couples therapy is spirituality, or more specifically, religion. Historically, people have turned to religion to be told who to marry, and while for many cultures this is no longer the case, our religion and spirituality can nonetheless lead to divides between you and your partner – as well as your families.

Religion

Particularly if you come from a religious background, it can be difficult for your family to accept a partner who is of a different religion to you – or indeed, a partner for whom religion is not a big part of their life. But as the world becomes smaller and we embrace other cultures more and more, there is no guarantee we will fall in love with someone from our own race or religion.

When it comes to religion, its effect on a relationship goes deeper than simply determining whether or not you will attend church on Sunday. Religious beliefs can play a part in choosing how to raise children, how you relate to your family, how you celebrate holidays, and even where you live and work.

But interfaith relationships – or a relationship between a believer and an atheist – are not necessarily doomed to fail. Let's take a look at some of the ways to make it work:

Respect each other's beliefs

As we have touched on many times throughout this book, one of the key steps to overcoming any disagreement is respecting and understanding your partner's point of view. Remember, in this case, it's fine to agree to disagree – the important thing is that you are able to openly discuss your views with one another, without passing judgement. This is particularly crucial in the case of spirituality and religion, as those who identify strongly with a particular faith often attach a part of their identity to their beliefs. And by criticizing their faith, you are by extension, criticizing them.

Share in each other's religion

Back in Chapter Three we discussed the need for you and your partner to have both shared and individual interests. Your partner's religion can be an important place to practice this. While it is important to give your partner space to practice their religion as they see fit, you can create a deeper connection between the two of you by participating in his or her religion from time to time. Remember, you don't need to be a believer to be a respectful observer. Consider going to church, synagogue or mosque with your partner from time to time, or attending a religious celebration. This helps you understand your partner on a deeper level, and also goes a long way to show them you accept this intrinsic part of themselves. It can also be particularly beneficial if and when you have children – if your children choose to follow in your partner's religion, you want to be able to share in this aspect of their lives.

Allow time for your partner to adjust

Even if your partner seems particularly willing to embrace your religion and all it entails, allow them time to adjust to changes. Acknowledge that introducing him or her into a new religion can raise questions and cause him or her to feel unsettled. Give your partner time to adjust to any changes, and be there to answer their questions.

Accept that it could be a deal-breaker

Sometimes it may be necessary to acknowledge that, for the devoutly religious, a partner who does not share their beliefs can be a deal-breaker. If you find yourself being cast aside for your partner's religion, acknowledge that it is not about you, but rather about their deep-seated beliefs – beliefs that were in place long before you came along. In such a situation, do not try to change your partner's beliefs, as this can lead to long-term conflicts between both you and his or her family. Rather, respect their decision and move on.

Broader Spirituality

These days, many people have a broader view of spirituality than just religion. Spirituality can encompass our relationship with the universe and/or our higher self, our relationship with the planet, and our beliefs surrounding the human soul, along with many other things.

And while it is not necessary to share the same spiritual beliefs with your partner, when you explore your spirituality together, it can lead to a deeper connection at all levels.

Increasing our spiritual connection with our partner

To increase the spiritual connection between you and your partner, you must first be clear on what spirituality means to you. You must understand who you truly are and what you want in life.

To do this, take some time to reflect on the following questions:

- What are my beliefs regarding life in general?
- What do I believe in terms of spirituality and religion? How important are these elements in my life? How important are these elements in a relationship?
- What do I believe in regards to God, or a higher power?
- Am a devoted to a particular religion or spiritual path? How committed am I to this path? How important is it that my partner shares this path? How will the decisions I make in this area affect my family (and wider community)?

- What daily rituals do I have regarding prayer, devotion or meditation? How non-negotiable are these?

Once you have taken the time to truly understand your own thoughts surrounding these important issues, ask your partner the same questions. Be sure you understand not only the answers to his or her questions, but also the underlying reasons behind these answers. Sometimes, talking openly about these matters and understanding the reasons behind your partner's beliefs can be enough to truly deepen your spiritual connection.

If you and your partner have spiritual beliefs that align with one another's, you might consider designing a daily spiritual practice that you can both share. For example, you might choose to meditate together, at the beginning and/or end of the day. The simple act of sitting in silence together can be a wonderful way of deepening your connection.

What to do when your partner doesn't share your spirituality

But what do we do when spirituality plays a large part in our lives, yet it is not something that our partner values? For many couples, this can become as valid a point of conflict as those trying to build an interfaith relationship. And just like interfaith couples, one spiritual and one non-spiritual partner does not necessarily spell the end for the relationship.

Just as we discussed in the previous section, the key is respect and understand. Challenges can arise when one partner not only doesn't share their spouse's spirituality but fails to understand why they have such beliefs in the first place. They may seek to make fun of their partner's beliefs, seeing them as too "new age" or "fluffy."

But the steps outlined above to help interfaith couples navigate their relationship can also be applied in relationships in which there is one spiritual and non-spiritual partner.

If you are the spiritual partner, consider ways you can share elements of your spirituality with your spouse, without forcing them to alter their beliefs, or engage in anything that makes them uncomfortable. This may be something as simple as reading them a passage from your favorite spiritual book, or asking them to sit with you for a five-minute meditation.

If you are the non-spiritual partner, firstly acknowledge that your partner's spirituality likely makes up a large part of their identity. Recognise that, by mocking or criticizing their spiritual beliefs, you are mounting a personal attack on them. While you should not be expected to adopt your partner's beliefs or practices (unless of course you choose to), agreeing to learn more about their spirituality shows you accept and respect a key part of your loved one. This serves to deepen the connection between you and will encourage you both to share more of your lives with one another.

Exercises:

CHAPTER FOURTEEN: PROBLEMS FACED
BY SPECIFIC COUPLINGS

While many problems faced by couples are universal, some relationships such as those between young couples, age-gap couples or those separated by distance have their own unique challenges to overcome.

Often, being aware of the pitfalls of these relationships in an important first step in overcoming the challenges. So let's take a closer look:

Young Couples

Perhaps unsurprisingly, lack of maturity is the underlying cause behind many of the issues faced by young couples. Particularly for couples who find themselves married or cohabiting immediately after leaving the family home, the lack of life experience can lead to a number of challenges.

So what are some of the most common issues faced by young couples? And how should we go about solving them?

Finances

For many young people, lack of money is a simple fact of life. Lack of career experience or training can make it almost impossible to find a well-paid job. As a result, many young couples find it difficult to make ends meet.

Lack of money can be fertile grounds for conflict, particularly if marriage or cohabitation has led you to want to save for a deposit on a home, or another large item. The shift from enjoying a life without responsibilities to having to save everything can be hard to maintain. And when one partner falls off the wagon and spends more than they ought to, it can be an ongoing source of conflict. See Chapter Nine for advice on managing financial disagreements.

Dealing with each other's family

For many couples, accepting their in-laws as part of the family can be a big challenge. This can be especially prominent at holidays, or other occasions when you would normally spend time with your family. Suddenly you have to make time for your partner's family as well. But remember, your in-laws are a very important part of your partner's life; and as such, they should become equally important to you.

If issues arise between you and your in-laws, it is crucial that you and your partner work through them together. Never ask your partner to choose between you and his or her family. Wherever possible, communicate any grievances directly with your in-laws, rather than having your spouse speak to them on your behalf.

Receiving unwanted advice from your partner's parents can be another source of conflict. If you find yourself in this situation, remind yourself that your in-laws only want the best for you and your partner, and their advice comes from a good place.

Finally, accept that, while your own parents must love you unconditionally, the same does not apply for your in-laws. The relationship between you and them will naturally be different to the relationship you have with your own family. Approach this sometimes-difficult situation with maturity, kindness, and a sense of humor. Remember how important your partner's family is to them – and how important your partner is to you.

Conflicts over household chores

Many young couples spend their days working, so there's little surprise that there is often conflict over household chores at the end of the day. To avoid petty disagreements spiraling out of control, try assigning each of you with set chores throughout the week, in the same manner you might do in a family or house-share arrangement. Sure, it might be less than romantic, but it will put an end to petty disagreements that can cause damage to your relationship.

Age-Gap Couples

Couples with a sizeable age gap can face a number of unique problems. While these relationships can be challenging, they can also be extremely rewarding. Having an understanding of the potential problems that may be faced in such a relationship can help couples smooth the road ahead:

Concern from family and friends

While you and your partner might be madly in love, those looking in from the outside – such as family and friends – can be prone to expressing concern over the validity, or suitability of the relationship. Lack of family support is sadly all too common in relationships with a twenty-year-plus gap.

If you find yourself in this situation, do your best to hear out the concerns of your family and friends, without criticizing them or immediately shutting down their arguments. Remember, they only want the best for you, and are concerned about your well-being. Once you have heard them out, ask yourself if any of their concerns are valid. Acknowledge that you have heard and taken on board their concerns, answering any questions in a clear and calm manner. This helps your loved ones feel heard, which is often all that is needed to gain their acceptance. If this is not the case, and you are committed to making your new partnership work, it may be in your best interests to take a step back from any toxic friendships and family members for a while.

Blended families

When you and/or your partner have children from previous relationships, creating a blended family can be a challenge – even without a sizeable age gap. But this challenge can be magnified in age-gap couples, specifically when existing children may be close in age to their parent's new spouse.

When it comes to facing this challenge, the first step is to be realistic. You should not be expected to fall in love with your partner's children instantly, nor should you expect them to instantly love you. Obviously, this is also true when it comes to your partner and your children. But it is nonetheless important that everyone involved works together to define boundaries and consequences together. For example, make it clear to everyone concerned that respect is non-negotiable.

Above all, be patient, with both yourself, your partner and any children involved. Recognize that this is a life-changing situation that will take some time for everyone to adjust to. Be open with your spouse about how you are feeling, and encourage the children to do the same.

The decision of whether to have more children

This is obviously a crucial question that should be considered by any couple, but it can be more pressing in an age-gap coupling, especially when one partner has already raised a family of their own, while the other has not.

Before making a commitment to each other, ensure you discuss this important matter with your partner. If the woman is the older partner, it may be necessary for her partner to accept that having more children is simply not an option. Alternatively, you might consider adoption, fostering, IVF or surrogacy. Whatever the case, it is important for both partners to be as open and honest as possible, not only with their partner, but also with themselves. If there is a need to compromise on this issue, is it a compromise you are willing to make?

Financial issues

Just like young couples, age-gap couples often face their own unique challenges when it comes to their financial situation. In age gap couples, it is likely that the older partner will be more established financially, than the younger. This imbalance can lead to conflict over who owns what, power struggles and/or feelings of inadequacy.

For age-gap couples, it is also important to consider how the older partner's retirement will affect the couple, as it will likely happen many years before their younger partner is in the same situation.

In such scenarios, the most beneficial course of action can be to visit a financial advisor and make a financial plan, outlining steps on how to move forward, with the minimum amount of conflict. Also see Chapter Nine for further information on managing financial disagreements.

Your lives going in different directions

While of course couples of any age can grow apart, this conflict is common among age-gap couples. Often, the older partner feels as though they have moved past the stage in their life that their younger spouse is in; for example, they might no longer wish to go out and party, or might be happier at home instead of travelling the world. This kind of divide can leave both partners feeling alone.

The key here is to address the situation as soon as it arises. Don't leave the conflict unspoken. Are their compromises you can both make in order to become a more active part of each other's lives? Or are you simply moving in too different a direction from each other to make this work? If this is the case, it is better to know sooner rather than later, before conflict and unhappiness becomes a part of everyday life.

Long Distance Relationships

Long distance relationships are never easy. Many people claim they can never work, and as such, will warn you away from becoming too committed to your partner. But if you are dedicated to making things work, anything is possible. Let's take a look at some of the key challenges faced by long-distance couples, along with tips for overcoming the challenges:

Loneliness

Being apart from your loved one on a regular basis can lead to loneliness and isolation, especially if you cannot just pick up the phone whenever you want due to time differences or other factors. Going out with your friends and their partners can heighten this sense of loneliness, making you miss your loved one even more deeply.

To overcome this, be sure to make plenty of time for your own interests and friends. Remember, your relationship is just one aspect of who you are, and keeping busy with other areas of your life will help keep loneliness at bay.

Communicating obsessively

While it may seem odd, overcommunicating is a key issue that arises between long-distance couples. Many feel that, to compensate for the physical distance, they must be in touch with their partner constantly, bombarding them with messages or phone calls throughout the day. But this behavior comes across as clingy and, bizarre as it may seem, can actually cause your partner to crave more distance between you. By all means, keep in touch each day, but there is no need to let your partner know you are thinking of them every five minutes. Sometimes, less is more.

Lack of physical contact

Not being able to touch your partner is undoubtedly one of the hardest things about being in a long-distance relationship. Human contact – both sexual and non-sexual – is both a physical and emotional need.

While you are unable to connect physically with your partner, you can connect emotionally. Keep the attraction alive through playful messages, innuendo and phone sex.

Finally, choose to see the positive side of the situation. While couples are unlikely to choose to go into a long-distance relationships unless they absolutely have to, the situation can give rise to a number of positives. Not only does it allow you to each grow as your own person, long distance relationships are wonderful at showing you how you truly feel about your partner. If you find yourself growing more and more distant as time goes by, it's probably a sign that your partner is someone you don't necessarily need in your life. But on the other hand, it may teach you that you want to spend the rest of your life with this person, no matter the situation.

PART 3: SEEKING THE HELP OF
A PROFESSIONAL

Perhaps as you have gone through this book it has led you to believe your relationship cannot survive without the proper professional help. If so, congratulations on taking the important first step of recognizing this is the case.

In this section of the book we will take a look at exactly what to expect in couples therapy, along with some of the common problems that arise during sessions.

Exercises:

CHAPTER FIFTEEN: WHAT TO EXPECT
IN COUPLES THERAPY

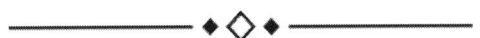

Usually conducted by a licensed marriage and relationship counsellor, couples therapy is a type of psychotherapy that allows partners to gain a deeper insight into the workings of their relationship and their behavior within it.

Couples therapy will usually begin with the therapist asking some basic questions about the relationship's history, along with interviewing each person about their family background, values and traditions.

Following this, the therapist will then work with the couple to determine the focus of the treatment and the goal(s) of the sessions.

Treatment generally consists of in-depth discussion, aimed at helping the couple gain insight into the way their behaviors affect the relationship's dynamics, helping them to understand what needs to be fixed, changed or improved.

Once insight has been gained, the next crucial step is making the necessary behavioral changes. To facilitate this, the therapist might assign the couple individual homework assignments, such as journal keeping, in order to keep track of the new skills they are adapting, as well as recognizing times when they slip back into their old, damaging ways.

For many couples, the end result of therapy is greater insight into the patterns of their relationship, as well as deeper emotional intelligence, and increased problem-solving abilities and communication.

Couples therapy can be beneficial for couples at any stage of their relationship, from those seeking premarital counseling, to long-term couples seeking to add a spark to their relationship. It is suitable for couples of any age, both gay and straight, who might be either dating, engaged or married. While couples therapy can be beneficial to assess the overall health of a relationship, it is most often used to solve conflicts arising from a certain area, such as infidelity, parenting, finances, sex, emotional distance or gambling.

While traditional couples therapy takes place, today's modern world is seeing a rise of alternative formats, such as online therapy and text therapy, in which the majority of treatment takes place in a written format.

Common Problems Arising in Couples Therapy

Over the course of this book, we have addressed some of the most common issues seen by couples therapists, including financial difficulties, sexual issues and parenting disagreements. But beyond these specific issues, there are a number of pitfalls that can arise when a couple embarks on therapy. Let's take a look:

 One of the main problems arising from couples therapy is that it is viewed by many people as a last resort. It is often seen as something that partners turn to when they are unable to resolve conflicts on their own or have gone through a major relationship-affecting event such as infidelity.

Thanks to this view, most couples come to therapy too late. Many couples seek help when their relationship difficulties are already significantly entrenched. Research indicates that most couples have struggled for an average of six years before they finally decide to seek outside help. At this point in time, damaging behavior has already been entrenched and the bonds between the partners has been significantly weakened. There may also be a high level of resentment as a result of past hurts and disagreements.

This is not to say, however, that couples with deeply entrenched issues cannot work through them. But the earlier couples embrace treatment, the easier it will be to unravel the damaging behavior that has led to each issue.

Another problem arises when partners see couples therapy as their chance to "change" their partner. This difficulty often rears its head when one party enters treatment believing they are in the right and their partner is the problem. For therapy to be effective, it is crucial for both partners to openly examine their behavior and be open to making the necessary changes. Beginning a therapy session with pre-conceived notions of who is right and wrong can hinder the process and deepen the rift between you and your partner. Instead of placing blame at your partner's feet, be open to the possibility that you are both able to make changes to better the relationship as a whole.

CONCLUSION

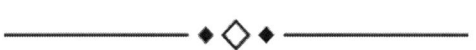

Each and every one of us who embarks on a romantic relationship will likely face one or more of the problems discussed in this book. It is human nature to disagree, and when we spend our lives so closely attached to another person, it is inevitable that conflict will arise.

But it is my hope that this book has shown you the way forward – shown you that, however damaged your relationship, it can be fixed.

As you have no doubt recognized, many of the solutions presented here revolve around one key element: open and honest communication. This is the essence of resolving all conflict, whether with your spouse, or anyone else in your life.

When we are open and honest, we are creating a space for effective communication; communication that can get to the heart of any issue – and then begin to resolve it.

So as you go forth and begin to mend the cracks in your relationship, focus on how you can keep the channels of communication with your loved one as open as possible. It will not always be easy – but it will be worth it.

BONUS CHAPTER

UNDERSTANDING INFIDELITY

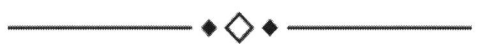

Infidelity is not a rare occurrence. Statistics demonstrate that 55% of adults have committed this fraud at some point. The question is, what preceded the infidelity? Can marriage or relationships survive infidelity? Even when both partners want to reconcile, can infidelity be forgiven? Is it possible to continue a life together?

Infidelity has its roots in many different factors, both in the relationship, and on the personal plane. There is always a warning, a sense that something is wrong. But that doesn't justify the infidelity. There are always problems that precede the cheating. So, the most common problems that precede fraud are all very similar, however, the first thing you will notice is the absence of a strong emotional connection. That connection may never have existed, or, alternatively, collapsed over time, because the couple paid insufficient attention to their differences or to the problems in their relationship. Infidelity is often a symptom of repressed dissatisfaction, unresolved conflicts, lack of communication, trying to find the passion, understanding, tenderness or love they don't receive in the relationship or the marriage.

This is the first problem, my friend—if something is bothering your partner the honest and preferred course of action is to talk about that problem. Infidelity is not an option.

The partner who chose to cheat reflexively places the fault on his/her partner. This, of course, is at least an acknowledgment that someone is being hurt. While most people have the opportunity to cheat, they overcome that urge, knowing that they will live with that truth for the rest of their life. Imagine having kids and cheating your partner. How will that affect them. Ultimately, the children suffer because someone decides to be selfish. Does that seem right to you? Of course not; it cannot be right. That is an example of pure selfishness. Do you understand the thought process of a person prone to infidelity?

Infidelity also is often a consequence of the loss of self-esteem, or a symptom of entering into a "mid-life crisis", or the result of a partner questioning the details of their past life—including work, career, and marriage.

When the fraud is revealed, the trust disappears, weakening the emotional and sexual attachment of the partner. Disbelief and the shock of discovery are universal reactions. Sadness, depression, negative self-worth, and intense anger toward the partner who committed fraud are typical feelings that accompany such a crisis. Even those who have had doubts become distraught when their worst fears are realised. At the moment of discovery, each partner reacts strongly, yet differently. In the first days and weeks, both are overwhelmed with feelings of tremendous loss, guilt, and shame. A cheated partner may react with tears, even rage. The situation may manifest in physical reactions, such as nausea, headache, sleeping and eating problems. On the other hand, the partner who has committed the infidelity often has a feeling of shame, remorse for what has been done, and a fear that the cheated partner will not forgive. The injured partner has lost the positive image of their life partner, and the belief in a secure, committed relationship. The partner who has committed infidelity has lost his/her secret love and also faces the potential loss of the marriage or the relationship.

Who is to blame here? We are not animals! We must resist this urge at any cost. It is very simple, my friend, when you love someone you don't hurt them. Once again, I will make this point—there is no justification for infidelity. If something doesn't suit you... leave the relationship. You will end things in a humane and proper way. Otherwise, you are nothing but a coward. As I said, every relationship is a highway. If you don't like it, take the next exit.

A person experiencing infidelity has lost trust in their partner, and they want to be assured that the relationship with the third party will terminate. They also want answers to questions regarding that relationship. A person has a long memory when it comes to a partner that had a love affair, that lied, that concealed infidelity, and they often visualize the details of the sexual relationship of the unfaithful partner. The partner who has committed fraud can respond with complete honesty, or with silence, because he/she is ashamed, and doesn't want to hurt the partner further. Whether or not reconciliation will occur depends on several factors, the most important being 1) the motivation to preserve the marriage or relationship, 2) the willingness to communicate honestly and solve problems, 3) the willingness to apologize and repent,and 4) the willingness to change, which sadly, is not always possible. That is the simple truth, so stop blaming yourself. Remember that the other party always had another option available.

1.1. You must know this as well

Infidelity does not mean that a relationship or marriage is "doomed". Although infidelity is one of the most difficult experiences of a loving life, it is possible to recover, and develop a relationship with greater trust, increased commitment, and deeper love. Couples can learn to successfully rebuild their relationship and make their relationship even stronger. Forgiveness is a difficult process, both individually and collectively. It takes work, on both the personal and the partnership level, to regain that lost confidence, and it requires both partners to exhibit a lot of patience.

1.2. What is essential?

To begin this process the transgressing partner must completely cease contact with the third party, and notify the deceived partner of any attempt by the e third party to contact him/ her. Honesty and loyalty will help to restore confidence in the relationship. In practice, it is useful for the deceived partner to know, in detail, the daily obligations and schedule of the unfaithful partner. This will remove all doubts regarding how the transgressing partner is spending his/her time.Serious conversations in which the reasons for forgiveness should be repeated and reinforced, and expressing sincere repentance for what has happened are obligatory. The apology of the partner who committed the fraud must be sincere and must include an acceptance of personal responsibility for the infidelity. Taking responsibility for your role is also very important to the process. This does not mean that both partners should bear equal responsibility for fraud, but rather identify the factors that influenced those events, so that they can prevent a similar occurence in the future. The best way to prevent infidelity is by constantly investing the time necessary to ensure the foundations of a marriage or relationship.

1.3. How serious is infidelity?

Apart from illness and death, nothing but infidelity creates such tremendous suffering. No matter how much time passes, perhaps as long as the marriage itself, there will still be difficulties in understanding why it happened. Why? How? We spinn in circles. This is not a healthy—ever.

People respond varied ways to the mention of infidelity, from bitter condemnation to resigned acceptance, to excitement and even approval. Infidelity may be ubiquitous, but how it is understood depends on the time and place of the drama. In the modern world, the love affair is primarily experienced through the damage it causes. It is always viewed through the lens of agony and the suffering caused by betrayal. The agony is that infidelity is not only causes a loss of confidence, but also the collapse of the high expectations of romantic love.

It is a shock that makes you question your past, your future, and your identity. The swirling emotions that emerge from the discovery of an affair can so overwhelm, that psychologists associate it with the symptoms of trauma: obsessive negative thoughts, excessive anxiety, numbness, alienation, unexplained anger, an uncontrollable panic.

The damage inflicted on a deceived partner is only one side of the story. Modern culture is much more sympathetic to injured partners. But not enough attention is paid to the meaning and motives of the affair, and what we can learn from it. The affair can teach us a lot about relationships or marriage—what we expect, what we think we want, and what rights we think we have. They reveal our personal and cultural views on love, lust, and commitment—views that have changed dramatically over the past one hundred years. Once again, if love exists—infidelity is definitely not an option.

1.4.   What is crucial?

We still want everything that the traditional family is supposed to provide—security, reputation, property, and children, but now, we also want our partner to love, want, and be interested in us. We should be the best of friends, and passionate lovers. We want our loved ones to offer us stability, security, predictability, and reliability. And we want it to last. What is the point of the story if your partner doesn't have the same perception of love? It's like trying to play a note on an old piano. You can hit the chords, but you will hear no music, my friend. That is a hammer hitting a string that doesn't exist.

1.5.   What is the point of everything?

At weddings, vows are made, and oaths to eternal love are sworn.Infidelity should never happen in the case of true love because all the reasons for it have been removed, and a perfect balance of freedom and a sense of security is achieved. But infidelity happens in good marriages and in bad. The freedom to leave the relationship or to divorce does not make the fraud obsolete. Since it is possible to leave, why do people cheat?

1.6.   And why do happy people cheat?

"Old wisdom" would say that adultery occurs when something is missing in the relationship or marriage, because if you have everything you need at home, as modern marriage promises, you should have no reason to go anywhere else to find happiness. Infidelity is a symptom of a failed relationship. So whatever the problem is, if you love someone, there are always two paths; the right path and the wrong path.

1.7.   Is infidelity in any way justified?

Theoretically, we all know that infidelity is immoral. However, there are situations where certain people will consider adultery to be justified, assuming that they are not the ones who are deceived, but it is very difficult to justify such an act.

Infidelity is a betrayal of a loved one's trust. More than a betrayal of trust, it is a betrayal of mutual respect. In principle, infidelity is a symptom of a pre-existing problem, but that hardly justifies it. You see where am going with this?

For example, a woman might consider infidelity as okay when a woman cheats on a man that is tormenting ther, especially if he cheated on her first. A man who cheats on his wife and gets away with it, may be considered by other, like-minded men, to be a hero of sorts. This is an example of pure hypocrisy. Another example is when one of the partners refuses to have sex for some reason or for no reason at all. After all, the partner being denied has to do something about his/ her natural needs. Really... trying to solve this problem with a loved one and/or complaining is not considered an acceptable way to meet those needs?

1.8.   And, what is the real justification?

The real justification doesn't exist. People cheat out of selfishness, because at that moment, they are satisfying their own needs (for sex, for attention, for feeding their ego), which, in the moment, is more important than whether it will hurtful to their loved one. It is also possible that they feel justified engaging in the fraud, because of some perceived hurt, but this is still not a valid excuse. If the relationship no longer works, it is better to end it than to cheat. If there is no sex in the relationship and one does not want to end the relationship, then those needs must go unfulfilled, thus avoiding harming the person you are in relationship with.

The shortest answer to the question of when is infidelity justified would be—never. There are other ways to deal with the problem that do not involve a betrayal of trust.

Made in the USA
Monee, IL
18 December 2020